ROGER WARREN BELIEVES THAT ANY MAN CAN BECOME DESIRABLE TO WOMEN . . .

if he is willing to put forth the necessary effort.

You may have a problem sexually satisfying the woman—or women—of your dreams. Or maybe you don't have a specific problem, but you lack the touch, the tone, the technique to really turn her on, to make you irresistible. Or maybe you just haven't found *her* yet and want to know how to go about it.

If you don't believe you're a master in bed, what you really want to know is How To Be An Erotic Man.

Roger Warren knows . . .

HOW TO BE
AN EROTIC MAN

Roger Warren

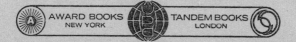

AWARD BOOKS
NEW YORK   TANDEM BOOKS
LONDON

Contents

HOW TO BE
AN EROTIC MAN

CHAPTER ONE

I Hate to Boast, But . . .

I'M NOT tall, dark, and handsome, and I don't have a playboy's bankroll. In fact, I'm quite average in appearance and, alas, average in income. Yet, for the past seven years since my graduation from college I have managed to date and go to bed with many attractive and desirable women.

I emphasize the fact that it is only recently that I have become successful with the fair sex, because while I was in high school and college I was something of a social flop. Oh, sure, I dated once in awhile and, on infrequent occasions, even managed to get laid. But chicks just didn't seem to find me exciting and, more often than not, my affairs with good-looking girls fizzled and died.

I like to think that my poor performance was mainly due to the fact that I didn't have a wealthy old man who gave me a big allowance and a sports car. That may have been part of it, but in being honest with myself I now must admit that I lacked the gentleness, self-assurance, and sexual creativity that women desire in men. In brief, I wasn't erotically sensuous.

Since my school days, I have learned that most men, regardless of what they look like or how much money they have, can be exciting, attractive and, perhaps, even irresistible to women. But, before this can happen there are several things they must first do to improve their attitudes, their knowledge of the psychology and physiology of females, and their understanding of their own sexual make-up. This information is not classified, nor is it innately endowed in a chosen few such as Casanova or Don Juan. On the contrary, the secrets of being erotically sensuous are just plain common sense and can be learned by observation and practice.

I guess I should tell you how I discovered this valuable information.

Soon after I started my first job at a New York advertising agency, I noticed that there were a few guys in the office who, while not being especially handsome, were dating the secretaries, models, and even some of the well-known actresses who did television commercials.

At first I thought these guys either had a load of bread or they were doing some couch-casting for the lucrative TV commercials. I soon found out these fellows were not earning a fortune and that none of them had anything to do with hiring the girls for ads and commercials. Being curious, and somewhat jealous, I asked Jerry, a copywriter who seemed very popular, how he managed to score with so many chicks.

"It's simple," Jerry began, "Women just seem to have a sixth sense. Call it ESP or feminine intuition, I really don't know. But whatever it is, chicks just naturally know which guys will be sensational in bed. Take it from me, it sure isn't money or looks, because I'm no Paul Newman and I usually have to borrow a few bucks to make it to payday."

Several weeks later, Jerry and I had lunch together and he went into detail about his sexual approach, his attitude toward women, his choice of clothing, and what he did to keep in shape. Through Jerry and a few other lady killers in the office, I gradually learned a few things about being erotically sensuous. I added to what these guys told me by reading up on the psychological and physiological aspects of male and female sexuality and by visiting a gynecologist friend to get a few "inside tips." I also did some serious thinking about my sex life up until then and made a conscious effort to get rid of my bad sexual habits and replace them with more effective techniques.

IT WORKED!

I hate to boast, but I'd bet you a week's wages that I go to bed with more women, more attractive, sexy, and exciting women in a month than most guys do in a year. Exactly how do I do it? To find out, you'll have to read the following chapters and practice what I preach. It works for me and it can work for you.

There's no reason in the world why you can't be THE EROTIC MAN.

CHAPTER TWO

You're Hurting Me! Be More Gentle

IF YOU want to prove how tough you are, play football or take karate lessons. Don't try to prove your masculinity in bed by crushing your chick's bones or by giving her black and blue marks as souvenirs of your love-making. Take it from me, most girls do not like the caveman approach. Of course, you may occasionally run across some women who really get turned on by bruises and welts—you know, the "Flagellate me and I'll follow you anywhere" kind. However, these ladies usually have emotional problems and generally make lousy bed partners because they are unable to find sexual gratification within the normal range of erotic experiences. By and large, most women like their men to be tender and gentle.

The importance of gentleness in sexual relations was first brought to my attention by Sandra, a girl I met at a cocktail party given by a well-known cosmetics firm she worked for. Sandy is a very attractive girl who, I later found out, really digs sex. As we sat and talked over our martinis, the topic of conversation quickly got around to relationships between men and women.

While we were telling each other about our personal ideas on man-woman relationships, Sandy told me quite offhandedly that she was bisexual. That is, she made it with girls as well as boys. When I asked her why, Sandy replied, "Let's face it. There are certain things you can do with a woman that you just can't do with a guy. I enjoy being in bed with men. I'm not a lesbian. But once in a while I go to bed with girls because . . . well, because they're more gentle than men. Lots of guys don't know how to treat a woman. They attack her, pinch her, and give her bear hugs that practically stop her circulation. God, you'd think they were making war not love. On the other hand, with a woman you don't have to worry about getting your breasts squeezed until they're black and blue. Women are more tender with each other. They know what it feels like to be hurt and they're more careful."

I thought about what Sandy had said, and I remembered the many times I was in bed with a girl who suddenly got turned off because I was being too rough. Think about it, you he-men. How many times has a chick said to you, "You're hurting me! Be more gentle." Being gentle is the first step toward becoming the erotic man.

How do you become gentle? Does gentleness mean being unmasculine? These are two questions that must be answered in order to assure both yourself and your chick more rewarding sexual experiences. Let's deal with the last question first.

Our culture tells a guy that to be a real man he must be aggressive, tough and dominant—especially in his relationships with women. To be less than these things meant you were a sissy or a fag. Unfortunately, this attitude stands between most men and complete sexual gratification.

Look at it this way. Men who are unsure about themselves as men—and there are lots of them—feel the need to prove their masculinity by relating to women with a "Me Tarzan, you Jane" attitude. They tell their women, "I'm the boss" and they try to emphasize their maleness by either consciously or unconsciously exhibiting their superior physical strength. On a harmless level this may be done when they offer to carry a bundle for a woman or when they courageously twist off the cap of an ornery Ketchup bottle. But, on a more dangerous level, there are some guys who must prove their maleness by beating their women or manhandling them before and during sexual intercourse in order to assert their masculinity. These guys, however, are only playing at being men, and the sexual act is required to bolster their weak egos. These guys have hang-ups about their masculinity, and their hang-ups block complete sexual gratification. If you don't believe me, just ask any psychoanalyst.

On the other hand, a man who is confident about his maleness and his ability to please chicks sees his woman as a partner in pleasure, a bed partner with whom he may freely exchange love, emotion, passion and feeling, without the need to feel superior to her. He feels equal to her and treats her in the way he himself would like to be treated. And, if he is normal, he wants tenderness and gentleness from his woman. In return he gives her warmth and gentleness.

Is this guy a sissy or a fag? If you think so, let me dare you to do this. When you come across a man who has the attitude toward women I've described, suggest to your wife or girl friend that she go out with him a few times. If he is a fag, you've got nothing to worry about. But, if he's a man who doesn't have to prove he's a man, your chick will start becoming more of a woman . . . with him.

What we have been talking about is a man's attitude toward women, and it is the attitude that must change before a guy can become gentle. Once this change of attitude has occurred, the next thing that must be learned is how to become physically gentle.

It is obvious that nature has made men taller, heavier and stronger than women, but society and culture also play a large part in making women more gentle than men. A young girl grows up using her hands for delicate work like sewing or cooking. A guy grows up using his hands to swing a baseball bat or fix a hotrod engine. When a female reaches her sexual maturity she has learned how to use her hands and her body in a way that will soothe and gently arouse men during sexual relations. A guy's first instinct is to approach love-making like a chiropractor manipulating a dislocated bone.

Men must learn to be physically gentle. To accomplish this, I have developed a series of Gentleness Exercises that I have used successfully to overcome my tendency to be rough with women. If you practice these exercises and apply them to your love-making, you'll find that your girl will be more responsive and passionate and, as a result, more able to please you.

GENTLENESS EXERCISE #1

Your hands can be used to drive a woman wild with sexual delight or to turn her off completely, depending on how you use them. It is most important for you to remember that as a man you probably have more strength than you realize. This lack of awareness is probably due to the fact that you haven't developed the sensitivity of touch that nature has placed in your fingertips. Because of this lack of development, many men find that in order to become sexually aroused, they must grab at a woman's body rather than caress it. They may achieve an erotic delight by doing this, but it's nothing like the pleasure they could achieve if their fingers and hands were attuned to the subtleties of the female anatomy. These subtleties can only be appreciated by gentle touching and firm but tender caressing.

To learn this "Magic Touch" you must teach your hands to recognize differences in tactile stimuli. To perform Gentleness Exercise #1, you must gather several items that have tactile qualities similar to the various erogenous areas of a woman's body. These items are:

A balloon filled with water
A small triangularly cut piece of fake fur
A round piece of foam rubber about the size of a small pillow

Now place the balloon in front of you and close your eyes. Using your right hand, squeeze it gently. Doesn't it feel like a breast? Women can become intensely aroused by having their breasts gently squeezed, but they can become turned off when pressure is applied. You'll know when you have the touch if you can squeeze the balloon without having it break. Practice alternately squeezing it and releasing it. Do this ten times. Now, repeat the exercise with your left hand.

Next, place the triangular piece of fake fur in front of you and close your eyes. Using the flat of your hand, press the fur very hard. Not much of a thrill, was it? Now, using your fingertips, pass your hand over the fur, barely touching it. Tickles a little? That's good. If that piece of fur were the pubic hairs of a woman's vaginal area, you'd be driving her out of her skin with the soft, gentle and erotic quality of your touch. Keep your eyes closed and continue passing your right hand lightly over the fur for about two minutes. Stop for a moment and then continue the exercise with your left hand.

I guess you're curious about that piece of foam

rubber. You're probably wondering how it fits in the gentleness exercise program. Well, let's satisfy that curiosity right now. Fold the foam rubber in half and slip a rubber band over each end so it stays folded. It doesn't take much imagination to realize that it feels very similar to a chick's backside. Now, you guys who really dig female posteriers, that is, you "ass men," pay close attention to this phase of Gentleness Exercise #1.

Many men think that female backsides are for pinching or grabbing. That's not always true. Sometimes they're for caressing. Once again, close your eyes and using both your hands, grab the rubber and squeeze it as hard as you can. If that were a chick's rear, you'd have her screaming in pain. Yet, that's what many guys do. Release your grip and pass the middle finger of your right hand gently over the opening of the fold so you can barely feel it. The soft roughness of the rubber is not unlike the flesh around the separation of a girl's buttocks.

Once your finger becomes receptive to the feel of this sensation you'll find that you'll often use the technique during foreplay and during intercourse when she is on top of you. Women find this stimulating, a lot more stimulating than having their rear ends grabbed as though they were fifty-pound sacks of flour.

This exercise should be practiced for five minutes with the middle finger of the right hand and five minutes with the middle finger of the left hand—which brings me to this point. To be a truly erotic man, you must be ambidextrous, at least as far as your love-making is concerned. If you are right-handed you may find there are times when your right hand is not in a position to perform the sensual touching you may desire. Therefore, you should be able to accomplish this equally well with your left hand. (Of course, this is equally true for left-handed men.)

I strongly emphasize that each of the Gentleness Exercises be practiced with both hands.

GENTLENESS EXERCISE #2

One of the most frequently practiced techniques for arousing women during sexual foreplay is for men to place their middle fingers inside the vagina and use them to stimulate the clitoris. If done correctly, fingering, as it is commonly known, can be a great erotic turn-on for both the gal and the guy. However, if done clumsily or roughly, fingering can be a sexual turn-off for women.

Many men who desire to arouse their women with this technique jam their fingers into the vaginal opening and proceed to rub the clitoris as though they were scratching a mosquito bite. While the damp warmth of the vaginal cavity may be exciting to guys, the harsh and insensitive use of their fingers may be painful to their women. To avoid this, I advise the following two-step exercise:

1. Press your lips back over your teeth and open your mouth about a quarter of an inch. If you do

this correctly, your mouth should have a tactile sensation similar to that of the outer lips of the vagina. Now, using the middle finger of your right hand, gradually slide your finger into your mouth between your lips and along your tongue until it reaches the back of your mouth. Hold it there a second or two and then slowly draw it out. You will be able to tell if you are being gentle by the feel of your finger against your lips and tongue.

Practice this exercise with your right hand until you are satisfied that you have reached the absolute maximum of your gentleness, then repeat the exercise with your left hand. Remember also that the slowness with which you do it is very important. Any slob can stick his finger into a vagina, but only an erotic man can do it slowly, dramatically and with feeling.

2. Once your finger is inside the vagina, your obvious purpose is to tenderly manipulate the clitoris so that your chick totally blows her mind. To achieve the proper technique for clitoral massage, fold your right middle finger back until it touches the heel of your palm. Then place a small round object such as a bead or a B-B shot between your middle finger and hand. Then practice rolling the round object for five minutes. The same finger motion you use in this exercise should be used to "roll" the tip of the clitoris. Remember, practice also with the left hand.

One thing more before we leave the topic of fingering. Always make certain that your fingernails are cut short and evenly. Long or jagged nails can hurt a woman's delicate sexual mechanism.

GENTLENESS EXERCISE #3

Several women have told me they can tell if a guy is going to be good in bed by the way he undresses them. Let me tell you about a discussion I had with a young lady I met while on vacation in Acapulco. Her name was Denise, she was from Los Angeles, and she was absolutely lovely. She was also married. Denise had come to Acapulco for a week to get away from her husband. I introduced myself to her at the poolside one afternoon and took her out to dinner that evening. Later we went back to my room and had one of the greatest passion sessions I had ever experienced. When it was over, Denise said, "That was fantastic! When I met you this afternoon I thought you'd be good in bed, but when you started taking my clothes off, I didn't think anymore. I knew. Some guys are real clods when they undress a woman. They fumble with buttons and hooks, they try to pull off your clothes, and more often than not they wind up tearing your blouse. Then there are the other guys, like you, who are really sexy about the way they undess you. They do it gently without tugging and pulling. Like I said, when you took my clothes off I knew you'd be a good lover and I was right!"

What Denise didn't know was that just a few short months before I was one of those clods she was talking about. Honestly, I often made a fool of myself when I tried to unbutton a girl's blouse or unhook her bra. I felt so clumsy, so cloddish, so unsexy as I fumbled with her clothing. One afternoon I discussed this problem with one of my buddies at work, and he suggested that I develop my finger dexterity by practicing with buttons, hooks and snaps at home. I took his advice and, as a result, developed the following set of exercises which can teach any guy how to disrobe his chick gently, quickly and sensuously. To practice these exercises, you'll need the following items:

> A button-front shirt or blouse
> A pair of slacks with a side or front zipper
> A bra

The first thing to do is unbutton and button the shirt several times with both hands. Next, button and unbutton the shirt with your right hand ONLY. Then, close your eyes and unbutton and button the shirt with your right hand. Practice the one-handed technique until you are proficient. Repeat these steps using your left hand. You might also practice buttoning and unbuttoning your own shirt one-handed so you'll be able to slip out of your own clothes more adroitly.

For the next phase of this set of gentleness exercises, place the slacks in front of you and practice zipping and unzipping the fly a few times with both hands. You'd be surprised at the number of guys who can't manage a zipper that's not on their own pants. When you have practiced with two hands for a while, use only your right hand to work the zipper. Then—you guessed it—do it with your eyes closed. When you become a right-handed zipper expert, teach your left hand what your right hand knows.

Finally, we come to the bra . . . the downfall of mankind. How many times have you struggled with one of those infernal things only to give up in frustration? Well, don't become discouraged. If man can reach the Moon, man can remove a bra. It only takes a little practice.

Place a bra on the table in front of you and examine the hooks as though you were Houdini examining an intricate lock. Then, slowly and deliberately, fasten and unfasten it. When you can do this easily, close your eyes and practice some more. No peeking! After you do it several times you'll find it's really no trouble at all. When you're making it with a chick and you take off her bra in no time flat, she'll mark you down in her book as a real pro. Incidentally, I do not recommend trying to undo a bra with one hand. Take it from me, it's damn near impossible.

GENTLENESS EXERCISE #4

Good old Dr. Sigmund Freud—the man who fired the first shot in the sexual revolution—explained in his theory of psychosexual development that human beings go through a stage in their infancy known as the oral stage during which they derive pleasurable impulses from sucking and biting. Freud went on to say that normal people grew out of the oral stage while neurotic people became fixated at this stage. Well, there must be an awful lot of neurotics around because oral sex has become the "in" thing. In fact, oral sex is so popular that I've devoted the entirety of Chapter Six to discussing various oral-erotic techniques. But for the present I think we should concern ourselves with overcoming certain oral-aggressive traits that keep many guys from being truly erotic men.

Ear nibbling, breast nibbling and other forms of nibbling are very important parts of the erotic man's bag of sexual tricks. However, too many guys confuse nibbling with gnawing. Instead of tasting a girl's body like a gourmet sampling a souffle, they go after her anatomy like a hungry dog on a bone. Remember, the areas of a girl's body you will be nibbling are extremely sensitive, and a sharp bite can be so painful that she may turn off entirely.

The following exercise will help you develop control of your mouth muscles so that your bite will be gentle yet passionate.

First, place your thumb about halfway into your mouth and bite down very gently. Then, move your lower set of choppers from side to side. Most men bite down, this is wrong. The side-to-side movement is more stimulating to women and it causes no pain. Now, as you are moving your jaw, circle your thumb with your tongue. Once you have coordinated the movement of your teeth and tongue you will have the perfect gentle mouth action that can be sensuously applied to almost any erogenously sensitive zones of your girl's body.

GENTLENESS EXERCISE #5

We come to the last and perhaps most important gentleness exercise: the control of the penis. Depending on how you use it, your penis can be either a vehicle of pleasure or an instrument of torture for both you and your girl. The problem with many guys is that they just can't wait to get inside their woman. Whether she's ready or not, they just force their erections into her vagina and think they're getting laid.

Well, buddy, that's not all there is to it. There is a right time and a wrong time to enter a woman, and there is a right way and a wrong way to do it. The right time is after a sufficient period of sexual foreplay so that she is "loosened"; that is, so that her vaginal muscles are relaxed and her vagina is lubricated by internal secretions. Less technically, this simply means that it would be best for you to "play around" for about five or ten minutes before beginning intercourse.

Now for the correct method for entering a woman. This involves a five-step exercise which, if practiced correctly, should make you a very desirable lover.

Step 1. Remove all your clothing and raise an erection. You may do this by either playing with yourself or by reading a horny book or by looking at a nudie magazine.

Step 2. Place the folded piece of foam rubber you used in Gentleness Exercise #1 on your bed with the open part of the fold facing upward. Then kneel in front of the foam rubber.

Step 3. Keeping your knees on the bed, lean forward slowly until your palms are resting on the bed and the weight of the upper part of your body is supported by your arms. Using only the muscles of your back, thrust your erection forward until the head of your penis enters the open part of the fold. Keep it there for a few seconds and then withdraw it. Repeat this several times. The purpose of this phase of the exercise is to develop your ability to test whether or not your chick is ready to receive your penis. If she is, the head of your penis would slip into her vagina easily without requiring the weight of your body to force it in.

Step 4. Maintaining the position described in Step 3, gently thrust your penis forward again, but this time allow about half of your erection to be covered by the rubber. Then, after a second or two, slowly withdraw it. This is an excellent teasing technique that women go wild over.

Step 5. Now that you have tested your chick's readiness, given her a taste of what it's going to be like and started to drive her crazy, it's time you got down to business. Slowly bring your erection forward as you did in Steps 3 and 4. Then gradually move your knees back and bend your arms until you are lying flat on top of the foam rubber. By doing this when you are actually making love, you'll avoid the thing that women hate—pouncing your weight down all of a sudden without giving your body the opportunity to find its optimum weight distribution on hers.

If all these exercises seem like a lot of unnecessary trouble, believe me, you won't regret it. The pleasure and reward you'll get from being a gentle and considerate lover will more than compensate for the time and effort you've spent on perfecting your gentleness techniques.

CHAPTER THREE

In and Out in Five Minutes

How Many of you guys remember the first time you got laid? I do. It was simultaneously the most exciting and the most disappointing event of my young life. I was excited because I had heard so much about how fantastic it was to make it with a chick. I had waited a long time and when the occasion finally did present itself, I felt like an air force cadet about to get his wings. Then suddenly it was all over.

Sure, it felt good, but not a whole hell of a lot better than masturbating. The girl, who was also getting her wings, and I told each other how great it was, but I was exaggerating and I suspect she was too. I guess we were both a little disappointed because it just didn't turn out to be all we thought it would be. Why didn't it? The answer is simply that we didn't do it long enough. I was excited—very excited—and it didn't take three minutes before I ejaculated. She didn't have nearly enough time to have an orgasm and I felt as though I had a wet dream.

Does that sound like a familiar story? Well, for lots of men, men who are not getting laid for the first time but for the hundredth time, that story remains true. For these guys their whole concept of balling amounts to in-and-out-in-five-minutes. Granted it provides a guy with physical sexual relief, but not with total erotic fulfillment. And it does nothing for the chick except make her feel frustrated. No doubt you've heard about women who go to psychiatrists thinking there's something emotionally wrong with them because they seldom, if ever, experience orgasm. Often there's nothing wrong with them, and it turns out that their husbands are not able to maintain an erection long enough to bring these women to the point of orgasm.

As a case in point, let me tell you about Sheila, a twenty-five-year-old divorcee whom I met through a mutual friend. When Sheila was eighteen, she had never engaged in more than light petting. She was a virgin until her honeymoon night. Her marriage ended five years later. There were many reasons for Sheila's divorce, and one of them had to do with sex.

"For five years I never had an orgasm," Sheila said. "Can you imagine that? Five years! Stanley—he's my former husband—just used to pounce himself down on top of me and we'd do it. A couple of minutes later he'd come and I'd be left high and dry. I guess Stan was just selfish about sex as he was about almost everything. He just didn't care if I enjoyed myself as long as he got his satisfaction. Since my divorce I've met lots of other men who really *care* if I enjoy myself in bed. They know how to control themselves so that they don't come until I'm ready to have my orgasm."

Sheila was quiet for a moment and then she added, "You know, I'm really sorry that I married so young. I should have waited and had a few affairs with different men. If I had had some experience, I never would have married my husband because I would have known what a lousy lover he was."

Do you see yourself in Stanley's place? If you do, you'd better do something about it quick. With the women's liberation movement and the waning of the double standard, women are going to feel as free as men to change sex partners if they aren't satisfied with the ones they have. Don't start worrying just yet. Let's examine the problem of the "quickie" and see what can be done about it.

Premature ejaculation is the term doctors use to identify the inability of men to control ejaculation until both partners have been able to derive complete erotic satisfaction from intercourse. There are several causes of premature ejaculation and, fortunately, most of them can be corrected either by men themselves or by doctors. Among these causes are heightened sexual sensitivity resulting from insufficient sexual relations, excessive masturbation, too frequent intercourse, prolonged periods of sexual foreplay and physical hypersensitivity of the penis.

Now that we have identified the problem and its causes, let's look into some cures. Through my own experience and through the recommendations of friends and doctors, I have put together the following list of techniques that may be used to control premature ejaculation. Perhaps one or several of these suggestions will be an answer to your problems.

TECHNIQUE #1

One of the most prevalent causes of premature ejaculation is insufficient sexual intercourse. Imagine a guy who hasn't been to bed with a chick in a long time, say two weeks or more. He finally finds a girl to go to bed with and they are lying naked next to each other. She touches him, he touches her. They kiss passionately and then he rolls on top of her. His erection enters her vagina and then ZAP. It's all over. He was so horny that he couldn't wait. Chances are the girl is not going to think very much of him as a lover. Now, all that could have been avoided by a very simple technique—masturbation. That's right, masturbation. Look, I'm a guy and you're a guy so let's say it like it is, jerking off. If you haven't made it with a chick in a long time, you're very easily aroused because you're physically and mentally in need of sexual gratification. Jerking off can alleviate some of that physical need.

Say you've got a date for Saturday night whom you know you're going to score with. The best thing for you to do is to jerk-off first thing Saturday morning. That way you'll be less excitable that night and more able to continue the act of intercourse for a longer period of time. A truly erotic man should never go to bed horny because horniness can make him blow his cool when the going gets hot. If I had to summarize this technique with an advertising slogan, I would probably say: "Jerking off shrinks horniness!"

TECHNIQUE #2

Some guys just can't help getting turned on by sex. As soon as they're with a chick and the going gets erotic, they become overly sensitive, and the result is premature ejaculation. My guess as to the cause of this would be that certain men have really been taken in by the mystique of sex and its forbiddenness. Then when they finally have intercourse, it's like a dream come true and they overreact.

I myself have never experienced this type of mental hypersensitivity, but guys who have tell me that the best way to overcome it is to read lots of dirty books, thumb through nudie magazines and go to X-rated movies. After a steady diet of this stuff, the forbidden nature of sexuality becomes less emotionally powerful and they can approach eroticism on a more psychologically even keel.

TECHNIQUE #3

Did you ever try to make love after you've done some heavy drinking? If you have, you know that at times it's impossible to even get an erection. I have found that drinking can be a cure for premature ejaculation. Now I'm not recommending that you spend an entire night drinking and then try to make it with your woman. What I am recommending is this: If you are a hypersensitive guy who comes before his chick has an orgasm, it would be a good idea to have a few drinks about an hour or so before you go to bed. A moderate amount of alcohol in your system will help to desensitize you enough so that you'll have more staying power and a greater ability to satisfy both yourself and your girl.

TECHNIQUE #4

There is a phenomenon which many men experience that I call "limited premature ejaculation." This means that these men can control themselves with most women but not with some. Over 90 percent of the cases of limited premature ejaculation that I've come across, both in my own experience and in the experiences of my friends, occur with women who are superfantastic at erotic foreplay. These chicks know how to use their hands, their lips and their tongues in such sensuous ways that they drive guys into erotic ecstacy long before actual intercourse begins. By the time their men begin coitus they're so hot that the mere entrance into the vagina is enough to make them come. What a letdown! It's like having a superb appetizer followed by a main course of pabulum.

I only know of one way to control limited premature ejaculation and that is to cut down on the preliminaries and get to the main course a little sooner. Any chick who is that good at arousing you deserves much more than a quick in-and-out session. She deserves a prolonged period of intercourse followed by an orgasm, and if you can't give it to her, there's always someone who can.

TECHNIQUE #5

Physiologically, certain men have naturally hyper-sensitive penises that are easily stimulated during sexual intercourse and cause premature ejaculation. If this is your problem, you might find the use of Nupercainal ointment is the solution. This ointment, which may be obtained at any drugstore without a prescription, is rubbed on the head of the penis and into the groove just below the head. After applying Nupercainal, you must wait about 40 minutes before having intercourse.

TECHNIQUE #6

If you prefer not to use ointment to control the supersensitivity of your penis, allow me to suggest an alternate method that isn't as good but does help a little.

It's a fact that most guys, married and unmarried, masturbate and chances are you do too. Now, there's nothing to be ashamed of. It's not sinful, it doesn't cause pimples and it may be useful in helping you control your premature ejaculation. It is possible to decrease the sensitivity of your penis by using a piece of rough cloth to masturbate with. A washcloth is perfect. If you jerk-off holding the cloth around your penis, the rubbing toughens the skin of the penis and makes it less sensitive.

TECHNIQUE #7

I told you earlier that excessive masturbation and too frequent intercourse can cause premature ejaculation. The technique for controlling premature ejaculation resulting from these conditions is simply to keep away from chicks for a while or to stop playing with yourself so much.

TECHNIQUE #8

Once you have gained control over ejaculation by using one or perhaps several methods described above, you are ready to practice the technique that will enable you to keep an erection and to keep screwing for hours. Yes, hours! The technique is called withdrawal, and it simply requires you to withdraw your penis when you feel you are about to lose control over your ejaculation. When you have done this, lie back on the bed for a few minutes, cool off and start all over again.

Women love this technique because it enables them to maintain their highest level of sexual excitement for a long period of time and, as a result, to have multiple orgasms. Any guy who has mastered the art of withdrawal will have his women coming back for more. I will say without qualification that withdrawal is the real mark of the truly erotic man.

If you find that these techniques are effective in

helping you control your tendency to ejaculate before both you and your chick have achieved total erotic satisfaction, I'm glad to have been of service. If, however, none of them work for you, it might be that you've got a problem that requires either medical or psychiatric attention. If that is the case, a few visits to the family doctor or a headshrinker may be what you need to become a better and more potent lover.

CHAPTER FOUR

An Erotic Man Shouldn't Have a Potbelly

GIRL WATCHING is easily the nation's leading male pastime, far surpassing baseball and pro football. Guys watch chicks in offices, on the streets and on the beaches. In fact, anywhere there's a good-looking chick, there's almost certain to be a guy glancing at her out of the corner of his eye, peering slyly at her over his newspaper or openly gaping at her. Women know this. That's why most chicks wouldn't dream of stepping out of the house without their hair, make-up and clothes in perfect order. And then there's the dieting! I know girls whose entire lives revolve around yogurt, poached eggs and melba toast. Do they suffer for health purposes? Not a one. They want to keep trim to keep the guys' eyes in their direction.

Now what about you men? Do you realize that while you're staring at a chick she may be looking back at you? What does she see? Does she see a flat, solid stomach or one that's hanging over the top of your pants? By the way, as terrible as a potbelly looks when you're dressed, it looks even worse when you've got your clothes off. What about those shoulders? Does a prospective female admirer see a set of square manly shoulders, or is she put off by saggy careless posture? And your arms. Are they the kind of arms a woman can feel safe and secure in, or are they flabby and weak?

Take a good long look at yourself in a full length mirror, first with your clothes on and then with them off. While you're examining that body of yours, ask yourself, "If I were a woman, would I find a build like mine sexy, manly and desirable?" If you can't objectively answer yes to that question, it's time you did something about getting yourself in shape. It really doesn't take much to do it. A little will power and determination, which you will have to provide, and a few simple exercises and diet hints, which I'll provide. Together we can give you the kind of body that women will like to be near; the kind of body that looks good with or without clothing; the kind of body that feels good . . . in bed!

Before we begin, I want to make it perfectly clear that you don't have to look like Mr. America to attract women. Actually, most chicks do not find inflated biceps, ape-like chests and bulging leg muscles particularly sexy. All that you really have to have is a body with a minimum of excess fat and muscles that have good tone. To get these you've simply got to exercise moderately and eat the right foods. Let's start with the exercises.

EXERCISE SET #1

I was always physically active in high school and college so I managed to stay in pretty good shape. But once I started working in an office I found myself putting on a few extra pounds and getting a little flabby around the middle. Several times I promised myself I would start exercising, but it wasn't until I received a not so subtle hint from Lauri, a photographic model I met at the ad agency, that I made up my mind to tighten up those loose stomach muscles. Lauri and I had finished making love in her apartment and we were stretched out nude on the sofa-bed in her living room. Lauri gave me the once-over and casually mentioned, "I hate it when men let themselves go. They expect women to stay trim and beautiful forever while they sit around getting jelly-bellies. There's nothing so unsexy as a guy with a soft mushy tummy."

I wasn't in that bad a shape, but perhaps Lauri was just giving me a warning. At any rate, I realized right then that an erotic man shouldn't have a potbelly. The next day I began the following set of sure-fire exercises for trimming down and tightening up the stomach.

1. The best way to start getting your midsection in shape is to do sit-ups. To do these, lie on your back with your arms stretched straight past your head. Then lift the trunk of your body, lean forward and touch your fingers to your toes. Your feet should remain on the floor. If you have

trouble keeping your feet down, have someone hold them for you. Do as many as you can each night for two weeks. These will prepare you for the next exercise.

2. Now that you've got your muscles limbered up, it's time to really get that stomach into shape. Lie on the floor just as you did in Step 1. Under your head place a heavy object, such as a ten-pound dumbbell and grasp the ends of it with your hands. Now slowly lift yourself as you did for the sit-ups. The added weight will cause your stomach muscles to work harder and get stronger. These sit-ups with weights should become a part of your daily routine. You'll find that after a while you will have no trouble at all doing them. At this time the amount of weight you are using should be increased.

A very important bonus of these exercises is the ability to achieve greater penetration of the woman. With fewer layers of fat belly flab between you and your chick, the closer you'll be able to get with less effort. This means that your erection will actually have increased your sexual potency, which will enable you to provide your woman with more erotic gratification.

EXERCISE SET #2

Your posture is very important. Good posture makes you look better and taller. It squares off your shoulders and makes you appear more masculine. Standing up straight with your shoulders erect instead of sagging also gives your clothes a better fit. And, most important, good posture is a great health aid.

When you allow your shoulders to droop, your chest becomes concave and that, in turn, limits the freedom of your lung expansion. When this happens, you naturally take in less air and you can easily become winded. This is devastating for the erotic man because it limits his intercourse endurance. How important is intercourse endurance? That is best answered by this story about Barry, an old and good buddy of mine.

Barry was fantastic when it came to attracting chicks but he was absolutely lousy at keeping them for more than a couple of weeks. Usually his girl friends split soon after they found out what a miserable lover he was. One day Barry confided to me, "It may sound strange, but when I'm with a really good chick, I lose my breath. I just can't seem to keep up with her. When this happens, I've got to do one of two things. Either I come right away and stop or I withdraw awhile and try to catch my breath. If I withdraw, I find that I'm so out of breath I can't raise a good hard-on."

Both Barry and I belonged to the same health club where we visited weekly for steam baths and rubdowns. While we were getting our massages, I mentioned Barry's problem to a masseur. Barry was embarrassed, but the masseur's answer was worth his embarrassment. He told us that cutting out smoking, doing lung development exercises, like jogging, and improving posture increased sexual vigor. Barry didn't smoke, but he also didn't exercise. And his posture was terrible. After hearing what the masseur said, Barry took up jogging and posture development exercises. The results, according to Barry, were unbelievable. His intercourse endurance increased as did the erotic gratification of his women. When I decided to write this book, I asked him which posture exercises he thought were the best. Barry recommended the following:

1. To perform this first exercise you'll need a broom or mop handle. Stand erect, shoulders back and feet spread slightly apart. Grasp the broom handle firmly behind your back. Keep your arms straight and lift the handle as far as you can, then slowly lower it. Be certain to keep your grasp on the handle as firm as possible, almost as though you were squeezing it. Repeat this ten times. As you do this exercise, you'll find several things happening. First, you'll feel your shoulders getting squarer and broader. Second, you'll feel your chest expanding. Last, you find a great difference in your lung capacity.

2. This next exercise is a familiar one. Stand erect and keep your shoulders back. Now, raise your arms to shoulder level and keep your palms flat and turned upward. Then, moving your arms from the shoulders, turn them in small counter-

clockwise circles. Do this twenty-five times, rest and then repeat the exercise, moving your arms in clockwise circles. If you do this exercise correctly you'll feel a definite pull across your upper back and shoulders. The best time to do this exercise is first thing in the morning.

These simple posture development exercises will make you look better in and out of clothing and do much to improve your lung capacity for greater physical endurance during sexual intercourse.

EXERCISE SET #3

"Put your arms around me honey, hold me tight." Remember that song? I grant you it's old, but the message is still as valid today as the day it was written. A woman wants a man whose arms are strong and protecting. When she's embraced by her man, a chick wants to feel secure and safe. Does your girl feel that way when you embrace her for a kiss or when you're making love? Or does she feel encased in a blob of blubber or surrounded by two tentacles of foam rubber? If your arms are flabby and weak, you'd better trim them down and harden them up. Here are some exercises to help you do it.

1. Chinning is one of the greatest ways of developing your arms. Most sporting goods stores have chinning bars that fit between doorposts. I recommend an investment in one of these bars. When

you start chinning, do only a few chins for the first few days and gradually increase the number as your strength and ability increase. In a very short period of time your biceps and forearm muscles will harden and the excess fat will disappear.

2. Another good exercise, for working up some extra arm muscle, is push-ups. Again, don't overdo it the first week. Let your arms and shoulders gradually work themselves into condition.

3. If you don't have time in your daily schedule to set aside for doing chins or push-ups, you might buy a rubber pocket gym. That is a section of rubber with a small handle at each end which, as the name implies, can be carried in your pocket, briefcase or lunchbox. You simply grasp the handles, hold the pocket gym at arms' length and stretch it as far and as often as you can. By doing this whenever you have a free minute or two, you'll strengthen your arm and shoulder muscles. I've also found that pocket gyms, used in the manner described, improve posture.

EXERCISE SET #4

Your lower back muscles are your "sex muscles" because you use them to thrust your erection forward during intercourse. Think about it for a second. When you're making love, which part of your body supplies the drive for your sex piston? That's right, the lower back. Do you know that low back pain is one of the most common medical complaints of men? One reason for this is that most guys just haven't had the opportunity or the need to develop this area of their bodies. The result is that many men are boring and unstimulating lovers because they are unable to execute varied and different intercourse positions that require good muscle tone in the lower back. In Chapter Eight we will discuss the various techniques of making love, but for the moment let's concern ourselves with getting those important sex muscles in the lower back into condition so that you'll have no trouble learning and using these wonderful and stimulating erotic positions.

The following exercise set is guaranteed to give you added strength, flexibility and staying power in your back region.

1. Lie in a supine position. Draw your knees up toward you until your feet are flat on the floor. Place your hands so that your palms are flat on the floor, fingers pointing forward and your arms about three inches from both sides of your body. Now, push up with your arms, arch your back and lift your midsection as high as possible without changing the position of your feet. Let yourself down slowly, rest and repeat the exercise properly. You'll feel it in the lower back.

2. Assume a push-up position. Only your toes and palms should be touching the floor. Keep

your back straight. Now, bring your midsection down so that only your pelvic area touches the floor. Do not bend your legs. Slowly bring yourself back to the original position. This exercise will stretch the lower back muscles in the direction opposite to that of exercise 1. By the way, isn't it remarkable how this exercise approximates the motions of intercourse?

These exercises should be done together so that you'll develop the proper upward thrust ability needed when your chick is in the female superior position, and the proper downward thrust ability in the conventional male superior position.

These four sets of exercises should keep you looking and feeling good while increasing your ability to perform well sexually. But muscle tone is only half the problem. The second half is developing good eating habits to help you lose that extra weight, keep yourself trim and maintain your sexual vigor. I've tried several diets that have succeeded in bringing down my weight. However, I soon went back to my old eating habits and put the weight right back on again. Most people diet that way—losing and gaining and losing and gaining. It's really a waste of time and effort and it's not particularly good for you to experience constant changes in your body weight. In addition, starvation diets can lessen your sexual desire and ability, and medical studies have shown that starvation will create nutritional difficulties which can bring about adverse physical changes in your genitals.

The problem then is to find a diet plan that will cause you to lose weight once and for all without denying your body the food substances it requires to perform the various functions . . . like sex.

A physician friend of mine recommended that I try the low-carbohydrate diet. He explained that according to this diet, calories are unimportant and what should be watched are the carbohydrates found in sugars and starches. I invested ninety-five cents in a paperback entitled *Dr. Carlton Fredericks' Low-Carbohydrate Diet* (Award Books) and browsed through it. I learned that all the carbohydrates I, or anyone else, needs is 60 grams a day. I followed the diet and lost 10 pounds the first month without denying myself any of the things I really dig . . . like booze. I also found that the low-carbohydrate plan can be used on a day-to-day basis as a maintenance diet. I heartily recommend the low-carbohydrate diet to you if you want to get slim and stay that way.

In addition to losing weight and keeping his body attractive, the erotic man should add certain things to his diet that will keep his sexual desire and ability strong. This is where my "Sex Diet Supplements" come in. There are two important nutritional elements that will supply you with erotic vigor. They are iodine and vitamin B. Your best nutritional source of iodine is shellfish and other seafoods. I've found that by eating seafood twice a week I'm able to keep myself ready, willing and able for *action* whenever it comes my way. By the way, seafood is low in carbohydrates.

A vitamin B deficiency in the male body causes an

increase in the estrogen level. Estrogens are female hormones and, believe it or not, we guys have them. A high estrogen level can substantially decrease a man's sexual desire and ability. To insure against this, I buy over-the-counter vitamin B pills and pop them a few times a week. Incidentally, a vitamin B deficiency in the female body has the opposite effect. When a girl is low in B vitamins, she feels a stronger sexual drive because her estrogen level is up. If your girl has been a little apathetic about sex lately, find out which foods are high in vitamin B content and keep her away from them.

Now that your body is in good shape, let's add to your attractiveness by dressing you up in clothes that are certain to make the chicks look twice. Chapter Sixteen will help you select the clothes that make the men who *make* women.

CHAPTER FIVE

When You Touch Me You Drive Me Crazy!

ONE OF THE biggest compliments a woman can give to a man is to tell him his touch drives her crazy, and to be a truly erotic man you *must* know just where and how to touch a woman so that every sensual nerve in her body responds. In Chapter Two we talked about ways to train your hands to be gentle and sensitive. In this chapter we'll discuss ways to put that training to use. What we are concerned with here is finding those areas of the female anatomy which, when expertly stimulated, arouse a strong sexual desire. Of course, most guys know *some* of these areas—the back of the neck and the ears are two examples—but there are many others. And knowing about these areas will make you more versatile and creative with your love-making and *much* more desirable to a woman.

The Palm

Believe it or not, a woman's palm is an erogenous area. The palm is highly sensitive and very respon-

49

sive to subtle stimulation. By gently moving your fingertips in a circular motion over your chick's palm, you will set off highly pleasing vibrations throughout her body. This is a great alternative to simple hand-holding and can be used in restaurants, theaters or any other place where more passionate touching is impossible. The sensations you cause by touching her palm are good previews of what she can expect from you in more intimate surroundings.

Between the Thumb and Forefinger

You'd really be surprised at just how responsive the area between the base of the thumb and the base of the forefinger can be. Try it on yourself. Lightly move your right index finger over this area of your left hand. Feels good? Well, it feels ten times as great to a girl whose hands are not quite as rough as yours are. Along with touching the palm, this adds variety to handholding.

The Inside of the Elbow

This is really dynamite! And it really turns chicks on . . . to you! By making gentle, small circular motions over the inside of the elbow, you can make your girl more relaxed and *less* resistant when you're ready to score.

The Ear

There are two ways to use a chick's ear to your sexual advantage: the wrong way and the right way.

The wrong way is to blow in it. To her it sounds like Hurricane Betsy and feels like an uncomfortable draft, neither of which are particularly enjoyable or sensuous. The right way is to stick your tongue in her ear and wet it slightly. Then cup your lips over her ear and gently inhale. That evaporates the wetness and produces a really out-of-sight sensation. In addition to this, gentle nibbling on the earlobe is something that most girls really go for, but—and I can't emphasize this too strongly—don't make the mistake many guys make and bite the earlobe. This is a real sexual turn-off.

The Back of the Neck

An airline stewardess once told me, "You've got no idea of how many guys really believe that if they blow on a girl's neck she'll follow them anywhere. I'd say that three out of five guys I come across think I'll melt if they exhale on the back of my neck. Sure, it feels good, but not nearly as good as the way a few guys do it." Those few guys this young lady is talking about are the real pros who add a little something extra and that is *licking* the back of the neck before blowing. Just the evaporation of saliva from the back of the neck increases the sensuousness of neck blowing.

The Breasts

If you think for one moment that you're going to turn an average woman into an empassioned nymph by grabbing her breasts, you're totally off base. A woman's breasts are perhaps the most sensitive and delicate parts of her body and they must be treated as such. To properly use your hands in this erogenous area, you begin by tenderly circling the nipple with your finger. Then softly roll the very tip of nipple between your thumb and forefinger. You'll know immediately if you're doing this right if your chick's nipples become firm and erect.

The next breast-touching technique is cupping your hands over your girl's breasts and alternately squeezing and releasing them. This should be done with a certain amount of firmness, but the one thing you must avoid is squeezing them to the point of hurting her. And above all, never never pinch a girl's breasts. This is probably the most painful and least erotic thing you can do.

The Pubic Hairs

A real pro with women is the guy who has mastered the art of "rumpling the short hairs erotically." The hair around the vagina covers a highly sensitive spot on a woman's body and you can make a chick melt in ecstacy if you follow this advice. Rest your hand between her legs and then, with your fingertips, lightly scratch the pubic hairs while barely touching the skin underneath. This touching technique comes with a 100 percent guarantee of satisfaction for her which means that she will be much more responsive to you.

The Backside

I mentioned in an earlier chapter that most men think of a girl's rear end as something to grab. And I also mentioned that grabbing is probably the worst thing you can do to a chick's ass if you want to start her sexual motor. However, there are two touching techniques specifically for the female backside that can keep your girl running in high gear.

> 1. When your partner in pleasure is lying on top of you, place both hands on the cheeks of her backside. Then slowly open and close your hands so that your fingertips move softly over her skin.

> 2. Again, with your girl in the superior sexual position, place your right hand, fingers spread apart, directly over the middle of her derriere and, with your middle finger, lightly tickle the area between her cheeks. Incidentally, you might also ask her to do this to you; it's really a fantastic feeling!

The Vagina

There's a world of difference between "fingering" a girl and sensuously using your fingers to produce within your chick a feeling second only to intercourse. Merely pushing your middle finger into her vagina and moving it around is an adolescent's idea of turning a girl on, whereas a man, an erotic man, goes about it in a more creative way. In the first place, you should begin by teasing your bed partner and make her anticipate the entrance of your finger. This is done by spreading her legs a bit and moving your middle finger slowly and gently around the outer lips of her vagina. After doing this for a minute or so, insert your finger about halfway and, very slowly, remove it. If you do this five or six times you'll have her out of her head in erotic anticipation. Now, insert your finger at the top of her vagina and slide it back until you reach the clitoris; this should feel like a small, hard bead. Gently massage it with your fingertip. At this point, your female friend should be a borderline nymphomaniac whose only desire is to give you one of the best love-making sessions you've ever experienced.

To add to your versatility as an "erotic voucher" you should know a few things about "sexual massages." There are few things that make a girl more relaxed before intercourse or more satisfied after intercourse than a massage; but not the bone-breaking type of rubdowns that guys are often inclined to give. If you make use of the following suggestions, you can give a chick a totally unforgettable erotic experience . . . an experience that will make her come back for more.

1. This massage is especially good after intercourse. Soak a soft cloth or towel with lukewarm water and rub your girl's back with it. Then,

before the water dries, fan her back with a dry towel or magazine. You'll get compliments on this one.

2. Put a small amount of cocoa butter on your fingers and lightly rub it all over your chick's body. This will feel good going on and also make her skin softer and thus more sensitive and responsive to your touch. This of course should be done before having intercourse.

3. The base of the neck and the spine can be massaged in order to reduce tensions and make your girl totally relaxed before sexual foreplay begins. Using your thumbs, apply a moderate amount of pressure to the base of the neck and, using a circular thumb motion, slowly work your way down to the base of her spine.

4. And now for the *pièce de résistance!* The fur glove! No massage makes a girl more eager for sex than a good rubdown with a fur glove. Believe me, I know. The technique I've found best is to begin the massage by softly rubbing the glove over a girl's legs. Then move up to her backside and then her back, concentrating mostly on the shoulder area. She'll love this—and you for doing it to her. And don't be shy, ask her to give you a rubdown with the fur glove. Incidentally, this massage also feels great after intercourse.

One last thing, don't overuse the massage technique. Erotic massaging is much more exciting if it's done when she doesn't expect it. Therefore, let a few passion sessions pass between each massage; that way you'll really have her looking forward to being with you.

CHAPTER SIX

You and Your Big Mouth

THERE'S A lot more a guy can do with his mouth than French kiss or bite a girl's earlobes. Today, the really in thing is oral sex and if you don't know how to do it, you're nowhere as far as many swinging chicks are concerned. Cunnilingus (eating), tongue baths, nibbling, licking and passion-biting are easily the most important kinds of foreplay an erotic man has in his sexual bag of tricks. There are any number of guys who become somewhat turned off at the thought of sticking their tongues inside; not infrequently, the vagina does have an odor. Well, chicks who dig sex appreciate this problem and many of them douche before making it while others use the so-called feminine hygiene sprays. And then there are some really thoughtful chicks who use *flavored* hygiene sprays and douches.

Although cunnilingus is probably the most frequent form of oral sex, there are several variations of oral eroticism that are available to guys who are willing to use a little imagination. And in the final analysis, it's your ability and readiness to discover and use original sex techniques that will make you the kind of man women want to be with. In all honesty, I must say that the oral-erotic techniques we're going to talk about are not my creations; they were passed on to me by a guy who is really an artist at love-making. In fact, he works in eroticism in the same way that Picasso works in oils. And, according to him, oral sex can be almost as exciting and enjoyable as actual intercourse.

Dessert

If your girl invites you for dinner one night, tell her that you'll bring the dessert. What you bring is a can of whipped cream. When dinner is over, she'll ask you what's for dessert and you say that *she* is. Sounds good already. Remove her clothes and put a dab of whipped cream on her nipples and a big swirl on her vagina. Hearty appetite!

The Before Intercourse Cocktail

Some guys like their wine straight, others like it on the rocks or with a twist of lemon. The way I prefer it is with or, I should say, on the chick I'm making it with. And more often than not, she likes it that way too. I call this the "Before Intercourse Cocktail" and it's very easy to make. Just dab a little wine on the nipples of a girl's breasts and slowly lick it off. It tastes wonderful and the licking combined with the evaporation of the alcohol in the wine feels wonderful to the girl.

Tongue Bath

This one is sure to blow her mind. Have your partner in pleasure lie on her stomach and, starting at her ankles, lick her legs. Then gently blow the area that you've licked. Repeat this on the cheeks of her backside and then slowly and sensuously lick her spine. Now, have her turn over and then lick the inside of her thighs near her vagina. By now she should be squirming with delight and ready to make it. But you're not finished yet. Lick her stomach—you'd be surprised at just how sensitive the stomach is—and then work your way up to her breasts. Now, have her reciprocate. After all, why should *she* have all the fun?

Eating

There are several different approaches to the art of cunnilingus and you can probably invent some of your own. The following few suggestions are good basic positions that leave many possibilities for experimentation.

THE FRONT APPROACH

Have your girl lie on her back with her legs spread. Then lick the inside of her thighs just as you did for the tongue bath. This is a good tease and warms her up for what follows. Now, run your tongue around the lips of her vagina a few times before inserting it into the vagina. When it is inside, move it back and forth as though you were licking an ice cream cone. In addition, you should fold your lips back over your teeth and open and close your mouth over the outside of the vagina. Add a little gentle blowing and you should have your chick at the point of orgasm.

THE REAR APPROACH

Ask your chick to kneel on the bed while you get underneath her. Place your hands around her backside and simply repeat what you did for the front approach only add the techniques of backside touching we talked about in the last chapter. By doing this, you'll have her going wild at both ends!

STRAWBERRY, CHERRY OR GRAPE

If you'd like to add a little flavoring or coloring when you eat your girl, put some jelly or preserves on your finger and rub it on and into her vagina. But be sure you lick it all up or things could get a little sticky later.

SIXTY-NINE

This position allows for simultaneous oral gratification. Lie on top of your chick with your mouth near her vagina and her mouth at your penis. Many "sexperts" prefer this position because it allows both the man and the woman to become excited together thus making them both ready for intercourse at the same time. Incidentally, if you want to be fancy, you can call the 69 position by its French name, *soixante-neuf*.

Nibbling

Your teeth can be used to add to your love-making abilities if you remember and use the techniques of "gentle biting" we practiced earlier. Women like the feeling of being gently "tasted" around their nipples, earlobes and vaginas. And this is done by nibbling and *not* by taking big bites. The best way to nibble your girl's nipples is to take the very tip of the nipple between your teeth and move it gently from side to side. At the same time your tongue should be pressed up against your teeth so that it touches the nipple, and it should move from side to side also. To add a little variety while nibbling, inhaling through your teeth will create a stimulating erotic sensation for your girl. Nibbling the earlobes is done essentially the same way. Again, remember to nibble and not to chew.

Nibbling the vagina differs slightly. Fold your lips back over your teeth, just as you did when you were preparing to eat your girl, and then kneel down alongside her. Spread her vagina apart and place your lips over the outer part of her vaginal lips and then firmly but gently press your lips together and move them back and forth. This technique may take a little practice to perfect, but take it from me, it's worth every second you spend practicing.

Passion Biting

There is a little sado-masochism in all of us, especially when passions are high. A lot of guys enjoy really sinking their teeth into some soft female flesh when they're making love, and, surprisingly, there are quite a few girls who like the pain. However, there are many chicks who definitely do not like passion biting. The best way to find out if you are with a girl who likes to be bitten hard is to slip in one good bite while you are in bed. This should be done only after extensive foreplay has made her very excited because certain chicks find that pain intensifies; then she's enjoying it. But do be careful not to do any real damage by biting too hard or too long.

May I offer some words of advice regarding oral sex? Many women, especially those newly initiated to modern methods of love-making may have an aversion to your placing your mouth on their vaginas. They may regard it as disgusting and unclean. The best thing to do in this case is to gradually introduce her to oral eroticism by nibbling, licking, biting or eating less "private" parts of her body. This process slowly conditions women to accept oral love-making. Then too, some girls may not object to your eating them, but they may not want to eat you. You can overcome this problem by gentle persuasion and by pointing out that it's not fair of her to expect you to provide all the pleasure for her while she does little to stimulate you. This line of reasoning works with most chicks. But if it doesn't work with your girl and if she simply refuses to perform oral sex with you, my advice is simply to find one who will. And that shouldn't be too difficult after you've become an erotic man.

CHAPTER SEVEN

There's More Than One Way To Do It

THERE WAS a time not too long ago when my idea of getting laid was lying on top of a chick and pumping away. But I've since learned that there's more than one way to do it, and *that* is the most important lesson an erotic man can learn.

Women can and do grow bored with guys whose sexual repertoire consists solely of the "male superior position," that is, the basic man-on-top, woman-underneath technique. When chicks make love they like variety, uniqueness and experimentation. And they love a man who shows imagination in finding new ways of pleasing them. Said one chick, "There are certain guys you just can't seem to get enough of. They make you look forward to balling because they always manage to come up with something new and different to turn you on and make you feel like a woman. I guess you'd say making love to them is an adventure. You never know what to expect."

Are *you* one of the guys she's talking about, or are you the typical man who does push-ups over a girl and then wonders why she's yawning from boredom rather than groaning with passion? If you fall into the last category, it's time we did something to get you out of your sexual rut. You may be surprised to learn that there are over a hundred different positions for making love; however, time and space do not permit my going into all of them here. What I can do, though, is offer you a cram course in some of the most interesting and pleasing positions for balling, which should allow you to pass any girl's erotic examination with flying colors. And after you've mastered these positions, you'll be able to ad lib here and there to create your own variations. With a little imagination you should be able to ball a chick twice a week for a year and never do it the same way twice.

VARIATIONS OF THE MALE SUPERIOR POSITION

KNEES UP

Lie on top of your chick, as you usually do, but have her raise her knees up and then firmly press them against your sides. This position allows for greater penetration of your penis into her vagina. To penetrate even deeper, place your hands under her backside and lift her midsection toward you.

LEGS CLOSED

Assume the male superior position. Instead of your girl spreading her legs, have her close them. This tightens her vagina around your penis—and take it from me, the sensation is terrific. You can spice this position up a bit by alternately contracting and loosening the muscles in your backside. This will make your penis "twitch" and girls love it. And, if your chick is really hip, she'll respond by contracting the muscles in her vagina and really blow your mind!

KNEELING

Have your girl lie on her back while you kneel between her legs. Then ask her to lock her legs around your waist. Holding her under her backside, thrust your penis forward. This technique allows for long leisurely strokes of your penis which, while not as intensely stimulating as the previous positions, allows you to have intercourse for a longer period of time. I especially recommend this one if you've got a chick who has been having trouble experiencing orgasm. The longer period of time spent in intercourse provides her with maximum opportunity to become sufficiently excited and reach climax.

ALTERNATING LEGS

Usually the standard male superior position means that the female has her legs spread while the man's legs are between hers. I've already mentioned one variation on this arrangement, another one is alternating legs. For this position simply have your chick keep her legs a little closer together than usual. You then keep your left leg between hers while your right leg rests alongside her left leg. In other words, one of her legs should be between yours, and one of yours should be between hers. This position allows you to enter your chick at a slight angle rather than straight ahead, thereby stimulating your penis and her vagina in a slightly different way.

VARIATIONS OF THE FEMALE SUPERIOR POSITION

BASIC FEMALE SUPERIOR POSITION

This simply means you lie on the bed while your girl lies on top of you. Of course, this also means that you must thrust upward, and that could take a few minutes of getting used to if you've never done it before. But usually the girl will meet you halfway. The first time I tried the basic female superior position I didn't care for it very much, but the second time I did it I enjoyed it as much as the male superior way. This position allows for several highly pleasing variations. Let's look at a few.

KNEELING

Lie on your back while your playmate kneels over your midsection. Thrust upward into her vagina. If you're a bit of a voyeur, as most men are, you'll love this position because you can watch your chick's body moving seductively while she's making love to you.

BACKWARD KNEELING

Again, lie on your back, but this time have your girl kneel over you with her back toward you. Chances are that you'll be unable to insert your penis into her, so ask her for a little help.

REVERSE FEMALE SUPERIOR POSITION

This is one of my favorites. While you're lying on your back, place your girl over you so that she's looking up at the ceiling. Then, after her legs are spread, insert your penis. This position allows for only minimum penetration, but your movements will stimulate the head of your penis as it's never been stimulated before. Some guys have told me that they've found it difficult to keep their penises from slipping out while using this intercourse technique, and I myself have found this to be true. The best way to overcome this is to have your girl hold it in place while you're making love. The greatest benefit of this position is that it allows you maximum use of your hands while balling. I suggest that you use this occasion to practice some touching techniques, especially around the breasts and the pubic hair area.

HINDSIGHT

All you ass men out there will love this one. Lying on your back, position your girl over you so that her legs are resting on your shoulders and her backside is facing you. Thrust upward. If you make love in this position you can watch her beautiful posterior in action. Try this technique once and you'll agree that sometimes hindsight is better than foresight.

BASIC REAR ENRTY

While your partner in pleasure is kneeling on the bed and resting her weight on her arms, kneel behind her and place your arms around her waist. Pulling her toward you, insert your penis. You can modify this position slightly by having your chick rest her head on her folded arms while you lean forward and rest your weight on your arms. Either way, the results are the same: delightful!

SIDE CAR

Both partners lie on their sides, with the male behind the female. The woman lifts her leg slightly as the male inserts his penis. This position is especially suited for prolonged sex. The male's strokes should be short and slow, while the female should keep her body moving in a slow sensuous rhythm.

STANDING REAR ENTRY

If you're getting a little tired of being in bed all the time, here's a position that offers a refreshing change of pace. Have your girl stand with her back toward you, then bend over and rest her hands on a table. Place your arms around her waist pull her toward you, inserting your penis as you do so. After your penis is inside her, you can ask her to close her legs and do some vaginal contractions.

SEX WHILE SITTING

SITTING BULL

Here's how to do it Indian style. Sit on the floor, a couch or, even better, a water bed if you have one. Fold your legs as though you were at a powwow and have your squaw sit on your lap facing you. Now you lean backward slightly, place your arms behind you and rest your weight on them. Then, with short forceful strokes, thrust your penis forward.

SEX IN A CHAIR

Find yourself a chair with no arms. Sit down and have your girl sit on your lap facing you. When using this position your chick will have to do most of the work because your movements will be limited by her weight on your body. An interesting variation of this position is having your partner sit on your lap with her back toward you. This variation allows for deep penetration and therefore makes it a really great sexual turn-on for your woman.

THE GREEK WAY

This usually gets people a little uptight. The thought of anal intercourse is, more often than not, distasteful to people who have never tried it. And indeed to some it may seem like a perversion, and that may be true if anal intercourse is used as the most frequent form of sexual gratification. However, if analism is used once in awhile as a variation in erotic relations, then there's nothing wrong with it. I've done it a few times and found it to be almost as gratifying as regular intercourse. The big problem with the so-called "Greek way" is that it can be painful to a chick who has never done it before. However, once she gets used to it, she'll probably like it because there are sensitive nerves in the anus that can be stimulated to create an orgasm in the woman.

If you would like to try making it this way, I suggest that you follow these instructions: (1) If possible, wear a condom. (2) Put Vaseline on your finger and insert it gently first; this will relax the woman. (3) Use the lubricant on your penis also, and proceed carefully, letting the woman control the penetration. (4) Proceed—with care—as you would during vaginal intercourse. (5) Never force entry; you may have to try this several times before you achieve success. (6) Wash your penis thoroughly after anal intercourse, especially if you intend to have vaginal intercourse.

Well, that about does it for our cram course in sex positions. Try them out, pick your favorites and don't be afraid to experiment with others. It would also be a good idea to ask your girl which positions she enjoyed the most. Then you'll know just what to do to please her and keep her coming back for more.

CHAPTER EIGHT

Don't Just Lie There— Say Something!

THE ONE thing that most men often overlook when they make love is the art of "erotic conversation"; that is, saying the right things at the right times in order to make their women feel more sensuous and thus more sexually responsive.

A complete approach to love-making means that all of the five senses should be brought into play. For example, many men get turned on by the odor of a seductive perfume, by the sight of black lace underclothes, by the touch of a woman's hand, or by hearing a woman whisper things in their ears. Well, women experience the same kind of excitement when their senses are aroused, and it's up to you as an erotic man to provide that total excitement.

Women, like men, love to hear nice things about themselves. Of course most guys know how to pay a girl a compliment by saying that they like her dress or that she looks especially attractive in her new hair-do. But this is Mickey Mouse stuff. It does nothing to make a woman feel like an erotically desirable and seductive siren. But let me tell you what will.

You can start out by saying things that let her know you're aware of her womanly qualities. For example, if you're dancing you might say, "There's something about the way you move your body that really turns me on." She'll smile at the compliment and then she'll slightly exaggerate her body movements so that you'll take even more notice.

Later on, when you're alone together, don't haul out the worn-out cliches like "You've got beautiful eyes," or "Your hands are soft and gentle." If you do you'll sound like something out of a 1945 movie. Be more direct. Tell her you love to feel her body respond to your touch. If you're touching her breasts, whisper, "It drives me crazy when your nipples get firm." And if she's teasing you with some wildly exciting foreplay say right out, "You know, you're a real bitch." That's not an insult. In a moment of passion there's nothing that makes a woman feel more sexy than being told she's a bitch.

A lot of chicks go out of their way to wear underclothes that will be exciting to men. And because they have been thoughtful enough to do this, you should reciprocate by telling them how fantastic they look. A girl in black lace bikini panties or a revealing bra feels sexy—there's a little bit of the exhibitionist in all chicks—and you can make her feel even more sexy by telling her that just looking at her drives you wild. Incidentally, I said this to one girl as she was walking around her apartment in her bra, panties, garter belt and black stockings. She smiled seductively and said, "You haven't seen anything yet." Then she turned on the record player and, to the rhythm of an acid rock song, sensuously removed the few things she had on. Needless to say, I became totally unglued. This just goes to prove what I've been telling you; if you say the perfect thing at the perfect time, you'll get some really out-of-sight results.

One idea that men have to get out of their heads is that using "four-letter" words in mixed company is vulgar. Of course, in many circumstances it is. But when you're alone and making love, a four-letter word properly used adds a little spice to the proceedings. You'd be amazed at a chick's response when you tell her that she's got fantastic tits, or that you love the feel of her ass. Such words have a very erotic sound; an almost forbidden sound and anything that is socially forbidden is very exciting.

Erotic conversation should be used before, during and after intercourse. When used before making love, erotic conversation is known as "verbal foreplay," and it's just as important as physical foreplay. In my experience, the most effective kind of verbal foreplay is telling your chick what you're going to do to her. Just before you begin to undress her whisper in her ear, "First I'm going to take off all your clothes. Then I'm going to lick you all over, and I mean *all* over. After that I'm going to give you a massage that's unlike anything you've ever had. Then, when you're so ready to make love that you can't wait another second, I'm going to put my cock all the way inside you." Now *that* gives a chick something to look forward to.

While you're making love you shouldn't expect your passion groans and an occasional "I love you" to communicate your feelings to your woman. You've got to be more imaginative than that. Tell her how wonderful it feels to be inside her, that her body feels fantastic next to yours, and that she's the most sensational bed partner you've ever had. Don't be afraid to lie a little; even if she isn't the greatest chick you've ever had, convince her that she is. She'll start believing it and, take it from me, her love-making abilities will improve enormously.

Then, after you've made love, build up her ego by complimenting her on her techniques. Knowing that she pleased you will make her want to please you again and again. Women like to be appreciated, especially as sex objects, because they have been taught that pleasing men is the most feminine thing they can do. So by telling her how much you enjoyed making love to her, you're making her feel more womanly. I learned this from a petite, hazel-eyed girl named Tara who said, "I really feel incomplete after making love when a guy just rolls over and takes a nap. I want to know if he enjoyed it as much as I did. I want him to say something like 'You really know how to screw.' I like love-making to end with an exclamation point, not a question mark."

CHAPTER NINE

There's Always a Time and a Place

AN EROTIC man, no matter how creative and imaginative his love-making techniques are and regardless of how sensuous and attractive his love partner is, might find that his bedtime activities are getting a little dull and unexciting. When this happens it might be his surroundings that are diffusing his sexual dynamite. Sure, it's great to have sexual relations in a comfortable bed, but that can become a little hackneyed after a while and you may need a change of scenery in order to put the excitement back into your erotic escapades. And this is not without its basis in scientific fact. There is a recognized form of psychotherapy called *milieu therapy* which operates on the theory that a person's problems may stem from certain conditions in his environment and that by getting away from that environment for a while an individual can overcome whatever personal problems are causing his hang-ups. Well, the same goes for sexual problems.

If your sexual relations have been less than great—

and they should *always* be great—it might not be *how* you're doing it, but *where* you're doing it that's causing your hang-ups.

Many guys have told me that simply by making it in a new place or at a different time than they usually make love, that they've improved their gratification and their chick's gratification 100 percent. And I can add my own amen to that. There are as many places to make love as you have the guts and imagination to find, but for openers let me tell you about some spots that my friends and I can personally vouch for.

Gilbert H. is a free-lance photographer who does a lot of work for ad agencies and women's magazines. One afternoon Gil was photographing a model in a secluded patch of woods. Before they could complete the shooting, a summer shower suddenly came. While waiting for the rain to stop they decided to make love. The girl thought they'd do it in Gil's station wagon, but Gil had another idea. They made love on the thick wet grass with the warm rain pouring over their bodies. Gil told me it was one of the most exhilarating experiences he'd ever had, and the model said it was really beautiful because she felt she was a part of nature. She explained that it was like being a nymph in the woods.

There's something about danger that quickens the sexual pulse, especially if that danger involves being discovered at any moment. I remember the first time I found myself in that kind of situation. A girl had invited me to her parents' beachhouse for the weekend so that we could be alone. Unfortunately, however, her parents decided at the last moment that they didn't want their "virginal" daughter to be alone with a man, so they just dropped in unexpectedly. That really blew it, or so I thought at first. That evening, while her folks were watching TV in the living room, we slipped away to her room and had ourselves a quickie. Her parents could have walked in at any moment and, knowing that, it heightened the intensity of the experience for the both of us. I don't know what I would have done if her mother or father *had* discovered us, no doubt it would have been just as embarrassing for them as it would have been for us.

I know one guy who really likes to live dangerously! He claims that the best quickie he'd ever had was with his boss's secretary in the supply room. Think of the office scandal that would have resulted if anyone had come in for supplies. This same guy also told me that he made it with a chick in a parking lot in Central Park during lunchtime when any one of the hundreds out for a noontime stroll could have peered into his car and gotten the shock of their lives.

A little dramatic and somewhat more romantic than a parking lot is the beach on a warm summer's night. There's nothing like it. The soft sand, the breeze and the stars create a perfect surrounding for some serious love-making. One thing—don't make love when you're wet from a moonlight swim. The sand sticks to you and it becomes a rather messy and uncomfortable experience.

If you can't find an interesting place for your intimate moments, your own apartment will do, provided you don't use the bedroom. For example, after dinner stretch out underneath the table and have each other for dessert. Or take a bath together and make it in the tub. Another good idea is to buy lots of giant overstuffed pillows and scatter them all over your apartment so that any room in the apartment can double as a bedroom.

If you want to create a really erotic atmosphere in your apartment, buy some strobe candles—candles that flicker when they burn—turn off the light, light up some incense and play some hard rock music real loud. This will change even the most unattractive apartment into a perfect environment for eroticism.

Impulse love-making ranks very high among guys who really know how to enjoy sex. Too many guys take the spontaneity and surprise out of sex by planning for it or by having relations only at certain times. One friend of mine insists on making it at the strangest moments, but he seems to prefer it that way. For instance, while out shopping with his girl friend one afternoon, the urge hit him. They checked into a hotel that wasn't concerned about their lack of baggage, enjoyed themselves for an hour, and then went back to shopping. It was unplanned and his girl was both surprised and delighted. As for myself, I also enjoy doing it at odd hours. The early morning is one of my favorite times. There's something about coming out of a sound sleep, slowly increasing your sexual desire, and then sharing a sunrise orgasm with a beautiful girl that puts you into a fantastic mood for the rest of the day.

An executive at my ad agency has his girl friend visit him during lunchtime. With his secretary at lunch, his telephone off the hook and the door to his inner office locked, this man finds that a few minutes of passion are a good way to break up a hectic day.

How About An Orgy?

The ultimate surroundings for a unique experience is to surround yourself with *other people*. That's right, invite your friends—your really hip friends— over for an orgy! Orgies are rapidly becoming very popular and for good reason. When you can see other people making it, when you can feel the hot atmosphere of a room full of erotic and sensuous people, your own passions are elevated to the boiling point. If you've never been to an orgy, let me tell you how to arrange one.

First, cover the floor with pillows and mattresses. The new water-filled mattresses are great for this purpose. Next, remove all your lightbulbs and replace them with low-watt, colored bulbs. You might also use a few flickering bulbs to get a psychedelic atmosphere. Incense, but not too much, is a must. Bowls of watermelon balls, orange slices, cherries and grapes that have been soaked in vodka for twenty-four hours should be within everyone's reach. And last of all, Turkish water pipes filled with red wine and amply packed with pot should be available if your friends are into the grass scene. Your record player should be stacked with sitar music, hard rock and modern jazz records. This atmosphere shoots down inhibitions and turns everyone into erotic people.

CHAPTER TEN

You Don't Need Spanish Fly

FOR THOUSANDS of years men have believed there were mystical and magical powers contained in certain foods and drugs that would make them more virile, increase their sexual endurance, spark the sexual potency that old age was extinguishing, or make their sex partners more desirous of intimate relations. On the whole, these foods and drugs have turned out to be useless as aphrodisiacs and, in certain cases, very harmful to those who used them. A brief overview of the attempt made by men to find the fountain of eroticism in mythical aphrodisiacs shows just how foolish and fruitless this search has been.

More than anything else, food has most often been the focus of the search for aphrodisiacs. Some people have believed that there was a great stimulating power in potatoes while others used tomatoes— once called love apples—to release their libido. Still others assumed that the shape of a particular fruit or vegetable gave it sexual powers. For example, carrots, because of their resemblance to the penis, were used to increase potency. While carrots probably did have a beneficial effect on the men who devoured them in an attempt to become more sensual, they did nothing to improve their qualities as lovers. Seafood has long been proclaimed as a sex-improving diet because of its high quantities of iron. These foods, however, are not aphrodisiacs in the sense that they heighten desire or performance, but only in the sense that they keep one's sexual equipment in good working order by improving one's general health.

Drugs have also played a prominent part in the history of aphrodisiacs. For many thousands of years, and even today, men in the Near East, especially those who feel their potency waning with age, used powdered rhinoceros horn as a sexual stimulant. A little closer to home the myth of the sexual power of morphine and cocaine derivatives has taken root in the drug subculture of today's youth. But the fact of the matter is that these powerful and dangerous drugs do not increase one's erotic capability but diminish it. Drug addicts are notorious for their inability to function sexually because of the loss of strength, vitality and physical health that so often accompanies drug use. This has a very detrimental effect on their sexual drive. Then too, there are those who believe that marijuana improves sexual relations, and this may be true. Grass does lower your inhibitions and place you in a receptive mood for having a good time, sexual or otherwise. However, grass may be more of a psychological than a physiological aphrodisiac.

Alcohol is often thought to be a sexual stimulant. This is partly true. In moderation, booze has a similar effect to pot in that it decreases inhibitions and makes you and your chick somewhat more permissive in your sexual behavior. On the other hand, if you get stinking drunk the alcohol tends to act as a depressant which decreases your sexual capabilities.

Now we come to the most fabled aphrodisiac of them all, Spanish fly, which incidentally, should be called Spanish beetle because it's made from dried beetles found in Southern Europe. Spanish fly is not a sexual stimulant but rather a chemical that inflames the urinary tract. The use of this drug, in both men and women, can be dangerous at the very least and perhaps fatal at the very worst.

A good part of the search for aphrodisiacs has not only been to make men more virile but also to seduce women. Well, if you're a truly erotic man you don't need Spanish fly or any other so-called aphrodisiac because *you* should be the catalyst that gets the female sexual chemistry going. Your attitude, your knowledge of how to please a woman and drive her wild with ecstasy, and your sexual creativeness should be all the aphrodisiac a woman needs. If you're looking for something outside yourself to turn chicks on, then you're not sure of yourself and perhaps even strongly doubt your own masculinity, and no drug—Spanish fly, alcohol or grass—is going to help you overcome these hang-ups.

While we've said that food is not an aphrodisiac, it does play an important part in your sex life. A well-balanced diet, along with moderate exercise, will go a long way toward helping you maintain your sexual desire and potency.

Aside from aphrodisiacs, men have also tried certain mechanical devices to make their chicks more passionate and responsive in bed. The device that most guys have heard of but few have actually seen is the "French tickler," a condom with short rubber protrusions near the front end. I'm not putting you on, the tickler *does* exist and there are some chicks who go for it. I came across an ad for French ticklers once in an underground newspaper and, out of curiosity, sent away for them. After I received the ticklers I examined them and kept them around the house as a conversation piece . . . I never really planned on using them. However, I did mention to one really wild chick that I had ticklers and she asked me to wear one the next time we made love. I did, and she started climbing the walls in delight. I didn't like the tickler, however, because it's so thick that I got virtually no feeling of being inside her. I recommend, though, that if you can locate French ticklers, buy them and use them once in awhile as a special treat for that infrequent girl who goes for them.

CHAPTER ELEVEN

What The Erotic Man Should Know About Birth Control

SEXUAL RELATIONS cannot be completely gratifying and totally enjoyable if either you or your chick have the slightest conscious or unconscious fear about an unwanted pregnancy. Nowadays, most erotically hip girls know about the various methods of birth control but you will undoubtedly run into quite a few who don't. If you aren't prepared with either a condom or good advice, there may be, at the very least, a hesitancy on the girl's part to be intimate with you or, at the very worst, you might find yourself shelling out later for an abortion or being slapped with a paternity suit. To forestall such unpleasant eventualities, it would be a good idea right now to examine the different birth control techniques and to compare their relative effectiveness and their convenience of use.

Sterilization

Don't get scared! I didn't say *castration*, I said sterilization which is done by a relatively simple

operation called a vasectomy that severs the vasa de-
ferentia which are the tubes that carry the sperm
to the seminal fluid. Sterilization does not reduce a
man's desire or ability to make love; it only does away
with his ability to impregnate women. There are
claims that this operation—which can be done in a
doctor's office—is reversible; however, most medical
authorities agree that for all practical purposes it is
permanent. Therefore, sterilization should only be
used by men who either have all the children they
want or by those who don't want children at all.

In the past year several of my married friends have
been sterilized and they have nothing but rave comments about it. One guy told me that his sex life has
improved because he's not bothered with thoughts
about having another child. Another fellow com-
mented that the sterilization has allowed him to be
more sexually spontaneous because now there's no
need for his wife to bother with her diaphragm when
the "urge" hits them. And still a third guy claims that
since his sterilization he's been getting a lot more
extramarital action because the girls he meets when
he's on business trips feel more at ease making it with
a married man knowing that there's no chance of
complications resulting from an empassioned one
night stand.

The Condom

A very effective method of contraception is the
condom or rubber, although it does have certain draw-

backs. Some men dislike it because they claim it lowers their erotic enjoyment by shielding the penis from direct contact with their women. And other guys find it somewhat of a hassle to put a rubber on because it interrupts their love-making. These two factors should be considered when you're choosing a method of contraception. Another thing to keep in mind is that although the condom is effective, it's not foolproof. It is possible to get a defective one that leaks or that might tear during intercourse. And it is not impossible for a condom to slip off while you're making love. Whenever I use a rubber I always test it before putting it on. This is done by blowing it up and checking it. I also test it afterwards by filling it full of water and checking for leaks. If a leak does develop, or if it slips off, the best thing to do is to have your chick douche immediately—although there is absolutely no guarantee that this will prevent pregnancy.

The effectiveness of the condom may be increased if you have your girl use a chemical spermicide such as vaginal foam or jelly. This precaution is a good back-up method in case the condom fails.

Withdrawal

Also known as *coitus interruptus,* withdrawal is another means some men employ to prevent pregnancy —but this is the least effective means of birth control. One drop of seminal fluid contains many, many sperm, any one of which can cause pregnancy. You can't get anywhere near the vagina to use this method and even your hands can carry sperm from the penis to the vagina. And besides this danger, you have to deal with the accompanying frustration of both you and your girl. Better to cool it when you're unprepared —and better luck next time.

The Pill

Oral contraceptives are probably the most widely used and most effective birth control techniques. The pill, used by women, does have many plusses. It is easy to use (one a day), it requires no interruptions in love-making, as do the condom and diaphragm, and there are no mechanical devices to fail or cause discomfort. There is one big minus, however, and that is that many women have reported adverse physical reactions while on the pill. If your chick is thinking about using an oral contraceptive, do her a favor and turn her on to a good gynecologist who can give her all the facts, pro and con, about the pill.

The Diaphragm

Most men have heard about this contraceptive device, but only a few have actually seen it. The diaphragm is a circluar piece of very thin rubber stretched across a spring. It is inserted into the vagina by a woman prior to intercourse and it is generally removed about eight to ten hours afterwards. Removing the diaphragm too early may result in pregnancy. A diaphragm is usually used with a spermicidal cream or jelly that seals any small openings between it and the walls of the vagina. Although it is a very effective method of birth control, the diaphragm can be bothersome to certain women who dislike taking the time to insert it. Unless the woman anticipates the love act in advance, she must interrupt the love-making sequence of foreplay to insert it. Sometimes a woman may just "forget" to insert it when her passions are aroused and she wants immediate gratification. This possibility may be circumvented if you have your girl insert her diaphragm several hours before you make love, even though spontaneity is gone.

The Intrauterine Device

More commonly known by its initials, IUD, this contraceptive device is made of plastic or metal and inserted, by a doctor, into the uterus. The benefits of the IUD are that once inserted, it can be worn for several years and it requires no preparation before intercourse. If a woman does wish to become pregnant, however, all she has to do is have her doctor remove it. The problem with the IUD is that it can be painful to wear for a woman who has never given birth. But it may be worthwhile trying because of its advantages.

Foams, Jellies and Sprays

There are many different types of spermicidal chemicals available but used alone they are not a very effective form of birth control. Although these chemicals are easy to use and therefore more convenient than the condom and diaphragm, vaginal creams, jellies and foams should generally be used in conjunction with a mechanical means of contraception.

The Rhythm Method

FORGET IT!

No matter what system of contraception you decide to use, remember that even the worst is better than none at all. However, the best thing for you to do is to speak to a qualified doctor or family planning organization and get filled in on all the particulars regarding birth control.

CHAPTER TWELVE

The Health Hazards of Sex

BEING AN erotic man doesn't mean making it with every chick you run into. In fact, it means the exact opposite. A guy who is sure of himself, who is secure in his masculinity and convinced of his ability to please women will usually prefer *quality* of sexual contact over *quantity* of sexual contact. On the other hand, a man with a Casanova Complex who feels he *must* score every night probably has grave personal doubts about his masculinity and uses frequent sexual contacts as a way of supporting his ego, alleviating his uncertainties about his attractiveness to women or demonstrating to himself and others that his manhood is intact. This is not an emotionally healthy situation and it can also be a physically unhealthy situation as well. The more sexual relations you have with chicks you don't much care about, the greater is the likelihood of getting venereal disease, and that can put any man, erotic or not, out of action for a while.

Many medical experts, who are by no means moralistic prudes, have said that the current Sexual Revolution has brought about a great increase in the incidence of VD, and they attribute this to promiscuity and lack of knowledge about venereal disease. Thus, reasonable cautiousness in selecting a partner in pleasure is one way of avoiding VD, and knowing some basic facts about these diseases is another. Let's talk about two of the most common varieties of venereal disease.

Gonorrhea, or "the clap" as it is commonly known, is an infection caused by an organism known as the *gonococcus* which is transferred during intimate contact. It can be passed from an infected woman to a man or from an infected man to a woman. If you contract the clap you'll see, after an incubation period of a few days to a week, a greenish-yellow discharge coming from your penis. This is usually accompanied by a burning sensation when your urinate. This symptom should be your warning to seek medical treatment as soon as possible. Your doctor will take a sample of the discharge and send it to a laboratory for analysis. If the results are positive—if you do have gonorrhea— he'll treat you with antibiotics. It pays to visit your doctor if you suspect that you've got the clap because left untreated, uncomfortable and serious complications may result. Too many guys think that having the clap is no more serious than having a bad cold. This is untrue. Gonorrhea can be dangerous.

Syphilis, also known as "The Syph," is transferred in the same way as gonorrhea. The early symptoms— lesions—generally appear at the point of infection, usually the penis. If you've been having oral or anal sex, however, these lesions could also appear around or in the mouth or anus. If these early signs appear, or if you suspect that the chick you've made love to is infected, visit your doctor for a blood test. This test will put your mind at ease if your fears about having the syph were unwarranted, or it will permit you to get treatment of the disease at an early stage. The cure for syphilis is antibiotics and it works in almost every case. Again, don't wait to contact your doctor because syphilis can develop into something more serious.

One myth that should be put to rest here is that VD can be transferred by contact with a toilet seat, towel or other object used by infected people. It cannot! VD is strictly a social disease and requires person-to-person contact.

Although I've never had the clap or syphilis, I've known several guys who have, and their unanimous opinion is to get medical treatment *fast*. Most of these guys said they were ashamed or embarrassed to visit a doctor because of the social stigma surrounding VD, but they didn't let that stop them. The slight amount of embarrassment you might suffer is nothing compared to the physical problems you'll suffer if you don't receive treatment. And another thing. You'd do both yourself and your chick a favor if you'd tell her that she might also have VD. This too can be embarrassing, but you have the moral responsibility to do it.

There are several *moderately* effective ways to keep yourself from contracting venereal disease. One we have already discussed, and that is not to be promiscuous. Another is to use a condom. Sure, this can take a lot of fun out of making love, but it's still a good idea—especially if you're making it with a chick whose "been around." It's also a good idea to wash your penis with soap and water after intercourse. And you might also recommend to your girl that she use an antiseptic douche. These are simple precautions, but they can go a long way toward keeping you—the erotic man—in action.

CHAPTER THIRTEEN

Orgasm!

EVERYTHING I'VE told you about being gentle in bed,
developing your sexual staying power, the sensuous
techniques for touching a woman, how to seductively
use your mouth for oral sex and the use of various
positions for intercourse has been directed to one
end: ORGASM! Without orgasm, sex is merely a
pleasant experience. If one partner experiences orgasm, then it becomes great. But if both achieve orgasm, then sex becomes fantastic! And that's what
being an erotic man is all about, making sex fantastic
for both you and your woman. However, the difficulty
is that a lot of men haven't the vaguest idea of what
an orgasm is or what to do to insure its occurrence.
So let's be scientific for a while and briefly discuss the
nature of orgasm.

Both the male and the female orgasm result from
a building up of libido or sexual energy during intimate contact. The muscles and nerves become tense
as this energy increases, and the sudden physical release of this erotic tension is the immensely pleasur-

able sensation known as orgasm. The orgasm is then followed by a period of relaxation. Aside from actual physical contact with a sex partner, orgasm can result either from masturbation or—mostly for males—from the sexual tension resulting from reading an erotic book, looking at provocative pictures or watching an X-rated film. Although men and women both go through the tension-release sequence of orgasm, there are many significant differences between the male and the female orgasm which you, as an erotic man, should know about in order to increase your girl's and your own probability of experiencing a fulfilling climax. Being gentlemen, we'll take the ladies first and examine the nature of the female orgasm.

HER ORGASM

Your woman's orgasm is not centered in the genital area as much as yours is. She feels the sensations of sexual tension release throughout her entire body, which means that her whole anatomy must be stimulated and aroused if a successful climax is to occur. Too often men concentrate their foreplay techniques on the vagina and breasts and ignore the other areas of the body. Of course, these two areas are *the* most sensitive; however, equal time should be spent erotically manipulating the thighs, legs, spine, ears, neck, backside and shoulders. Furthermore, women require a considerably longer period of foreplay than men before they are psychologically and physically prepared for orgasm. The worst thing you can do is enter your chick before she's ready. She won't enjoy making love as much, and you'll wear yourself out trying to bring her to the point of climax.

Even after extensive foreplay, your woman will need a relatively longer period of coitus than you will to achieve orgasm. The longer you can keep your erection firm and in action the greater is the likelihood that she'll experience an unforgettable orgasm. The techniques of sexual desensitization and withdrawal that we discussed in Chapter Three are useful here. And if you can keep yourself from shooting your load too early, you'll be able to give your woman multiple orgasms. If you can accomplish this feat, she'll never stop thinking about your qualities as a lover.

Aside from physical stimulation, women also require psychological stimulation in order to achieve orgasm. Many studies have shown that a large proportion of women have never experienced orgasm. On the whole, this may be attributed to the attitude our society has toward female sexuality. Our puritanical standards have indoctrinated women with the idea that if they enjoy the sexual act they are perverse tramps. Therefore, many women see sex as a necessary evil, something they must do in order to please their men. And even some of the more sexually liberated females are still affected by this thinking, and this may influence their ability to have orgasm. If you find that despite all your erotic tricks your girl is unable to have an orgasm, perhaps she's the victim of some prudish Victorian attitude. I once knew a girl with this type of hang-up. Her name was Janet, and I met her at a party given by a mutual acquaintance of ours. Janet and I dated several times after the party, but it wasn't until the third or fourth date that we were alone together. She didn't try to stop me from making advances and she didn't seem to mind going to bed with me. But that was it. She made love because she felt she had to make love, but she was a real cold fish about it. No passion, no orgasm. I asked her quite frankly if it was my fault that she didn't seem to be enjoying the relationship. She answered, "It's not you. I'm always like this. I want to make love, and I want to enjoy it. But there's something that keeps me from going all the way emotionally."

We talked for a while and Janet told me about her upbringing. She came from a very strict New England home where her mother had always emphasized the "proper" behavior for a lady. She was taught that sex is something only men like and that women who enjoy it are somehow immoral. Although living in New York for a year had liberalized her attitudes toward sex to the point where she did make it on occasions, she still had this unconscious hang-up that it was base and dirty and this kept her from experiencing climax. We got together for several rap sessions and talked about her feelings. The more she verbalized her old-fashioned attitudes the more she was able to see how ridiculous and wrong they were until one evening Janet experienced her first orgasm. It was simply a matter of letting go. And that should be one of your talents as an erotic man, showing chicks how to open up and let go of whatever problems are standing between them and total sexual fulfillment through orgasm.

YOUR ORGASM

We men really have a problem when it comes to getting the most enjoyment out of our sexual relations. In the first place all but a few guys are incapable of multiple orgasm, whereas most women can have several in a row. Being "oversexed," as we are, we tend to get hotter more quickly than women, which leaves us much less time to enjoy the build-up stages of intercourse before we achieve climax. And, once we have achieved orgasm, we come down from our sexual highs more rapidly than women. All this is the fault of our biological plumbing. The male orgasm is genital centered and we rely for orgasm on the discharge of semen. Once we have ejaculated, the sexual desire passes from us with the seminal fluid. Chicks, on the other hand, don't rely on bodily discharge for climax, which means they can keep going a lot longer than we can.

The trick is to control your seminal discharge long enough so that your woman can have her orgasm. We have gone into detail on this topic in Chapter Three and I suggest that you re-read that material. If you can abstain from shooting your load too quickly, not only will you provide your chick with more satisfaction, but you'll experience a more gratifying orgasm because you've waited and allowed the sexual tension to build to the point where you can't wait any longer. At that point you are psychologically and physically more able to appreciate the tension release of orgasm.

Once you have experienced a ringing climax, you'll probably feel like rolling off your chick and taking a nap. DON'T DO IT! As I've said, chicks come down more slowly than men and the one thing they hate is when a man comes and then withdraws and goes to sleep. Your woman will appreciate you much more if, after orgasm, you stay inside her and let your erection gradually shrink its way out of her vagina. The movement of your penis as it becomes smaller and smaller is very exciting to erotically aware women.

One last thing about orgasm. No matter how erotic you are or how good your chick is, you're *not* going to experience orgasm every time you make it. Orgasm depends on your frame of mind, the state of your health, and the strength of your sexual drive. All these are variables that can and do change from time to time and modify the quality of your overall sexuality. And the same thing goes for your woman. There may be times when she's just not prepared to put all her effort into making love. But don't be discouraged if you miss having an orgasm or producing one in your chick. Even erotic men slip up once in awhile.

CHAPTER FOURTEEN

Will She be Good in Bed?

How MANY times have you met a girl who really looked *sexsational*—you know, beautiful body, provocative clothes, sexy make-up—who later turned out to be as passionate as a clam and as erotically stimulating as a cold shower? Probably more times than you care to remember. The problem with us men is that we too often believe what we see. We live under the delusion that if a chick looks good she's going to be hot stuff in the sack. Well, as the song goes, it ain't necessarily so. There are any number of women who don't look like Raquel Welsh and who don't come on like a sex-starved nymphomaniac who, when the lights are out, can glow with sensuality.

Then there are chicks who look fantastic and talk a great game but that's as far as it goes. As an erotic man, you should be able to separate the winners from the losers and there are a few tricks that will help you do this. But let me say this, there's no sure-fire way of picking a dynamite playmate every time. No matter how good you are at spotting a phony or a tease, once in awhile one will slip through your defenses. The advice I'm offering, however, should improve your batting average so that you don't strike out too often when picking a partner in pleasure.

A woman's eyes are often the mirrors of her sexuality. There's a lot you can tell about a woman by the way she looks at you . . . if *you* know what to look for. Don't be fooled by the soft, watery, kitten-like stares that girls work so hard at perfecting. Chicks are smart and they know that men find this sexy. What you should notice about a woman's eyes is the way they move. Does she coyly give your body the once over? Does she look at you when you dance? Does she seem to undress you with her eyes? If the answer is yes, then you've probably got yourself an erotically aware female who knows what she's looking for in a man and who knows how to express her gratitude for finding it.

The way a woman touches you communicates a great deal about her abilities to please men. If she simply holds hands with you in the movies or across the table at a restaurant, then chances are she doesn't know how to use her fingers sensuously. But, if she tenderly strokes your palms, teasingly moves her fingers up your arm, or gently touches your fingertips, you can be almost certain that she's capable of putting her hands to good and pleasurable use when you're making love. When you're making out, beware of the girl who keeps her hands in one place. Chances are she'll do the same thing in bed. However, a chick who touches you all over, who enjoys feeling your body, and who occasionally digs her fingernails into your back is telling you something about her passionate nature.

Perhaps the best way to tell if a chick is going to be good in bed is by the way she kisses. A girl who closes her eyes and "puckers up" is sure to be a sexual drag. No doubt she's been watching too many old Doris Day movies and getting some pretty dumb ideas about sexual behavior. By the same token, watch out for the chicks who kiss you so hard that your teeth move backward. They're trying to *act* passionate and in bed they'll probably continue acting. Personally, I hate going to bed with a girl like that because I feel as though she's auditioning for a part in a movie rather than involving herself in the realities of making love.

The kind of kiss that should tell you you've found the right woman goes something like this. First she wets her lips a little. Then she gently presses her mouth against yours and perhaps seductively nibbles your lips. Next, her tongue slowly slips from her mouth to yours and moves lightly across your tongue and touches the roof of your mouth. While she's doing all this, her body is pulsating seductively against yours and her fingertips are lightly touching your neck, your ears and your hair. You don't need anyone to tell you that a chick who kisses like this is bound to be a winner.

For heaven's sake, watch out for girls who always

look like they've just come out of the beauty parlor or who spend a long time putting on make-up. While these chicks may look good, they usually turn out to be nothing in bed. In the first place they don't want you to get too passionate because you might ruin their hairdo or smudge their make-up. And in the second place the amount of time they spend making themselves look good should tell you they're probably self-centered and egotistical and therefore selfish lovers who couldn't care less whether or not you enjoy yourself. And be just as wary of women who talk in great detail about their sex lives. Frequently these chicks are sexual novices who have just "discovered" sex and haven't had much experience, or they're latent prudes who want to come on strong to attract men but who then turn-off under the covers.

One question that many guys have when picking a playmate is, "Should I make it with a virgin?" The answer depends on you and what you're looking for out of a sexual relationship. If you're the type of guy who enjoys teaching a woman about sex, if you don't mind putting up with a virgin's hesitancies about such things as oral eroticism, and if you want the knowledge of being the first man to give a chick her wings, then by all means look for an untouched flower. But if you like a woman who knows what she's doing, if you don't care where she learned what she knows, and if you're willing to learn a few new tricks yourself, then pick a playmate who has been around. One other thing, if you are after a virgin you might find that

she's hard to lose when you want to end the relationship. Chicks almost always get hung up over the first
guy they've made it with and saying good-bye to
them can be a very sticky affair.

CHAPTER FIFTEEN

Ethics and Morals

IT MAY seem strange to find a discussion of ethics and morals in a book that deals with the far-out kind of sexuality we've been talking about. But let me say this: *Morals have nothing to do with the sexual behavior of two consenting adults.* What I do in the privacy of my bedroom with a woman who chooses to be with me is no one's concern but our own. My concept of morality is that I've got the right to do as I damn well please just as long as I don't interfere with anyone else's right to do as they please. As far as I'm concerned, there's nothing more immoral than a person who attempts to set standards of personal and sexual behavior for others. Some people may accuse me of oversimplifying the topic of morality because I'm not making an allowance for the religious and social mores that govern sexual activity. That may be so; however, sex is a simple act of pleasure and there is no need for a complicated set of moral rules to regulate the activities of two people who get together to enjoy themselves.

What is important in sexuality are the ethics of the two sex partners in regard to each other. A successful sexual relationship not only depends on the ability of the man and woman to satisfy each other erotically, it also requires an understanding between them so that each knows what to expect from the other. What I'm about to say about my own code of sexual ethics is no more than a set of guidelines that I've established for myself and found useful in my dealings with women. You may ignore them, disagree with them, or adopt them as your own. The choice is yours. I'm merely passing them along to give you something to think about.

1. Never force your brand of sexuality on women who are unwilling or unready to accept it. Just because you happen to dig a certain style of making love doesn't mean that everyone else does. For example, if a woman is unwilling to perform oral sex on you, you shouldn't force her to do it. In this case, just do the things you can both agree on and make the best of it. Next time, find yourself a girl with the same sexual appetite as yours.

2. Never take advantage of a woman who is drunk or under the influence of drugs. I know any number of guys who literally force alcohol or other inhibition-reducing drugs into girls and then make it with them. If you need drugs in order to get women to make it with you, then

you're not really much of a man. And you're certainly not an erotic man.

3. Never fool around with underage chicks. Aside from the legal implications, there are also ethical implications. A young girl might not be psychologically prepared for adult sexuality and you could do her a great deal of emotional harm if you treat her in the same way that you'd treat an emotionally mature woman.

4. Always make sure that proper birth control precautions have been taken before you make love. Too many guys operate under the rule of "fuck 'em and forget 'em," meaning that anything that happens after he cuts out is the chick's problem. It's simply not fair to expect a woman to have an abortion or raise an out-of-wedlock child just because you couldn't take an extra minute or two to prevent conception.

5. Be honest. Don't promise a girl that you'll marry her in order to break down her resistance to having intercourse with you. Keep the relationship on the up-and-up. That way you'll avoid unnecessary emotional complications.

6. Don't screw and tell. There's nothing worse than a guy who shares intimate relations with a chick and then announces it to the world. Your sex life is your business and no one else need know about it.

7. Keep away from your friends' wives and girl friends. Fooling around with someone else's chick is the best way to lose a good friend and maybe even get a black eye in the bargain.

A good thing to keep in mind is that word gets around, and if you treat women badly you'll suffer in the end. A guy who gets a reputation for only being out for what he can get from women soon finds himself getting no women at all. It's good practice for an erotic man to keep his head straight about his ethical and moral responsibility to women. Remember, not only do chicks love a man who's a good bed partner, they also like a guy who treats them fairly. When it comes to being a successful ladies' man, good guys finish first.

CHAPTER SIXTEEN

An Erotic Man Should Dress the Part

Now THAT you act and and think like an erotic man, the next step in making yourself irresistible to women is learning how to look like an erotic man. Your clothing and personal grooming habits create the first impression that women have of you and, like it or not, first impressions are what women often use in separating desirable men from undesirable men.

You can be the most fantastic lover in bed, the greatest conversationalist at cocktail parties, or the nicest guy in the world and still get left at the starting gate if your physical appearance doesn't light a chick's fire. I'm not saying that you have to be handsome to attract women. Nor am I saying that you should have plastic surgery and come out looking like a movie star (however, I do know one guy who had a nose job which, he claims, improved his sex life 1,000 percent). What I am telling you is that your clothes, your hair style and your grooming communicate a good deal about you. If you look interesting, hip and sexually desirable, women will beat a path

111

to your bedroom. But, if you look like a creep, they'll beat you away with sticks.

Chicks are very clothes conscious, they learn about styles, fabrics and color coordination as part of their girlhood training in femininity. Attractive attire—on men or women—catches their eye. Sloppy, ill-fitting, and out-of-style threads also catches their eye and gives them something to laugh about when your back is turned.

Unless you've been hiding in a cave for the last five or six years, you must be aware that there's been a revolution in men's dress. The blue oxford button-down shirt, the narrow tie, the drab three-button suit, and the cordovan clodhoppers have yielded to bell bottom slacks, wide ties, flamboyant shirts, fringed vests, fitted suits and highly styled boots and shoes. And this is good news for men. Not every guy looks good in the same type of clothes. In the past the selection was limited and you were just out of luck if the current styles didn't suit you. But now you've got an almost endless variety and choice of clothes and hairstyles that highlight your good points and hide your not-so-good points.

CLOTHING

Dressing well is no more difficult than dressing poorly; the difference is simply knowing what to wear and what not to wear. In selecting a suit, a jacket, or a shirt you have to take these things into account:

YOUR BUILD

If you're short, avoid long suit and sport jackets. Wearing them will only accentuate your lack of height and make you look like one of the seven dwarfs. Husky or heavy men would do well to keep away from pinch-waisted jackets. A looser fitting garment won't draw as much attention to your midsection. It's also a good idea for overweight men to forget about wearing "hip hugger" slacks until they've lost a few inches.

Although the "natural" look is currently in vogue, it's not a bad idea for thin men to add a little extra padding to the shoulders of their jackets. It gives their clothing a nicer shape by helping to accentuate the tapered look that predominates in men's clothing.

YOUR COMPLEXION

Men with pale or sallow complexions do not look good in yellows or greens. Such colors make them seem as though they have terminal yellow jaundice. Reds, blues, oranges and other bright colors are good choices when buying shirts, while navy blue, dark gray and lively prints are recommended for suits and jackets.

If you've got a ruddy complexion, don't wear red. You'll only look like Santa Claus. And if you've got red hair *and* a ruddy complexion, green is not your color. Dark complexioned men should avoid somber-colored suits and dark shirts.

YOUR AGE

The younger you are, the more you can get away with in terms of dressing wild. But men entering their mid-thirties, unless they look much younger than they are, should temper their stylishness with a bit of restraint and moderation. There's nothing more ridiculous and pathetic than a middle-aged man dressed up like a teeny bopper.

A very important part of the revolution in men's clothing is the trend away from the formal and toward the informal. In times past it was required of a man taking a chick to a movie, party or to dinner to wear a tie and jacket. Nowadays, hip guys wear fancy vests and body shirts or turtleneck sweaters with form-fitting jackets. And even at "black tie affairs," black ties aren't being worn by fashion-conscious men. Instead, they're wearing wide and wild ties with colored shirts.

I could go on and on about the changes in men's fashions, but I think you've got the general idea. What it really means is: be an individual in your dress. Express yourself in what you wear. Throw convention to the wind and let yourself go. A good place to begin your own personal clothing revolution is in the pages of such magazines as *Gentlemen's Quarterly*, *Esquire* and *Playboy*. These publications carry ads for all that is new on the clothing scene and offer many valuable hints for selecting the threads that will help you come across as an erotic man.

PERSONAL GROOMING

HAIR

There's a big difference between a barber and a men's hair stylist. When you come out of a barber shop you look essentially the same as you did when you went in except that your hair is shorter and you smell from witch hazel. But when you emerge from a men's hair stylist, you look like a different man, and for more guys, that's an improvement. A good stylist charges more than a barber, but he does a lot more for your money and your appearance. He styles your hair to suit your face, he artistically hides those bald spots, and he performs all kinds of little tricks like covering up your Dumbo ears and rounding off your pointed head. A good-looking hair style gives a guy confidence in his appearance, and we all could use a little more of that.

Facial hair, notably beards, mustaches and sideburns are what's making news in male grooming. Women have told me that a beard gives certain men character, while a mustache changes an ordinary-looking guy into a suave and sophisticated man about town. And of course, sideburns go a long way toward making you look like you know what's happening. If your face can stand a little improvement, a beard or mustache may be just what you need. Your hair stylist has loads of suggestions as to the proper kinds of beards and mustaches for your type of face.

And now a few words for you guys afflicted with the curse of baldness. Unfortunately, the Yul Brynner look is out and the Tom Jones look is in. And that means that men with thinning or nonexistent hair are going to face difficulties in the pursuit of sexual happiness. But don't despair. There is hope. If you've got lots of money, patience, and time, a hair transplant isn't a bad idea. But if your bread is low, an investment in a good hairpiece will fill the bill. The great demand for men's hairpieces has made good rugs available at moderate prices. And with modern glues you can swim wearing your hairpiece, take a shower with your chick without it falling off, and even make love in it. I personally know several guys who wear rugs without ever arousing the suspicions of their chicks. However, I also know a couple of guys who have faced the embarrassing moment of having their hairpieces accidentally removed by overpassionate females while making love. But even then it wasn't too bad. It was dark and the chicks were having such a good time that they really didn't care whether or not these guys had a full head of hair.

FINGERNAILS

I never thought I'd live to see the day when I'd have a manicure. I've always considered men with manicured and lacquered nails somewhat foppish and unmasculine. That was until a buddy of mine insisted that I try it once. I did and, surprisingly, I liked it. I thought my hands looked good and, more important, chicks thought my hands looked good. Said one girl, "I hate men with uneven nails and overgrown cuticles. Their hands look sloppy and feel terrible when they touch you. But a guy with a good manicure is something else. His hands look kind of sexy, and they're nice to hold or be touched by." Since then I've had a manicure regularly, and I suggest you do the same.

GROOMING AIDS

There's a lot to be said about using heavy, greasy hair tonics, and it's all bad. There's nothing girls dislike more than running their delicate and sensitive fingers through a man's hair that's just had an STP oil treatment. There are many good greaseless hair grooming aids on the market that will keep your hair natural looking, in place and pleasant to touch. My particular favorite is men's hairspray. A light spray after combing my hair keeps it neat for a long time and makes it easy to touch up with a wet comb. Several of the better men's toiletry companies offer men's hairspray scented like their colognes and after-shave lotions. This is a great idea because it allows your hair to smell like the rest of you.

As long as I mentioned after-shave lotions and colognes, let me say a few more words about them. I've said several times in this book that a successful lover seduces a woman by stimulating all five of her senses, including the sense of smell. Just as you love the subtle and sexy odor of an alluring perfume, chicks like the masculine and clean odor of a good shaving lotion or men's cologne. So my advice is to buy several bottles of the *expensive* colognes and shaving lotions and wear a different one every day until your special girl comments that she prefers one over the other. Or, if you want to be more direct, simply ask her which cologne you should buy. The trick to using men's cologne or shaving lotions correctly is not only splash some on your face, but dilute a few drops with water and spread it over your entire body after you take a shower. Then, no matter where your chick is kissing, nibbling, or sucking you, your body will emit a pleasing masculine aroma.

And, most important of all, always use a deodorant or antiperspirant. No girl likes a man who smells bad.

UNDERCLOTHING

Do you like to see your chick in baggy bloomers or in sexy bikini panties? Of course, you prefer the panties. What man wouldn't? Well, let's put the shoe on the other foot. Does your chick want to see you in baggy boxer shorts or in well-fitting underwear? Again, the baggies get the negative vote. If your body is in reasonably good shape, you might consider buying some sexy male underwear and watching your girl's eyes sparkle with delight as you strip for action. I'm not kidding, many of the hip men's clothing stores sell fishnet undershirts and semi-bikini men's shorts. Believe me, they do turn chicks on, and I've found them to be a lot more comfortable than regular underclothes.

Before I give the "over and out" on the topic of men's clothing and grooming, let me re-emphasize one point: no matter how much time you spend perfecting your oral love-making techniques, no matter how many sexual positions you know, and no matter how gentle you can be with women, you're not going to get a chance to use your sexual skills if your appearance turns chicks off. If you've spent this much time and effort to become an erotic man, you might as well go all the way and insure yourself of success. So get rid of those drab out-of-date duds—give them to the Salvation Army—and get yourself some hip, swinging, way-out threads. You'll look great and feel great, and the chicks won't leave you alone.

CHAPTER SEVENTEEN

Can A Married Man Be An Erotic Man?

The Answer is definitely YES! There's absolutely no reason why a married man shouldn't use his sexual creativity and imagination with his wife. It's no secret that sex is one of the single most important aspects of marriage and that if a husband and wife have a poor sexual relationship they'll probably also have a poor marital relationship. Any number of married people have told me that the best way to keep a marriage alive, happy and mutually satisfying to both husband and wife is by avoiding the dullness of stereotyped love-making. Couples who can discover new erotic turn-ons together, who avoid the cliches of love-making and who treat sex as a dynamic part of their relationship will be much more compatible than husbands and wives who view sex merely as an obligation forced upon them by the marital contract.

The problem that keeps many men from enjoying full erotic satisfaction with their wives is the ridiculous notion that it's somehow improper or immoral to engage in the same kind of sexual practices with their wives as they did with the girls they dated when they were single. That's a lot of crap! Just because a woman is married doesn't make her any less of a female, and that means she has the same desires and drives as a single girl. There's nothing wrong with having oral sex with your wife or experimenting together with new sexual positions or making love on the floor of the living room or in the back seat of the car. When you do these things, you make her feel like a sex goddess. She knows that you appreciate her not only as a cook or housekeeper or working wife, but also as a seductive, exciting and desirable partner in pleasure.

Whenever the topic of sex and marriage comes up, the question of extramarital relations can't be avoided. Even guys with fantastic sex lives at home once in awhile get the desire to stray from the marriage bed. In fact, studies show that over 90 percent of married men have at least one extramarital affair. Realistically then, the question shouldn't be "Should I have an affair?" but "How do I go about having an affair?"

In a world built on honesty and a better knowledge of human sexual behavior, the answer would simply be to tell your wife that tonight instead of going bowling, you're going to spend the evening with a chick who means no more to you than a good lay, a simple sexual change of pace. However, we haven't progressed far enough socially and psychologically for this to happen—if indeed it is progress. So what we're left with is finding ways to have a little outside stimulation without getting caught. Although I'm not married, I did ask some of my married friends how they went about having affairs while avoiding discovery. Their answers are summarized in the following list.

Nine Rules for the Married Man

1. Never have an affair with a woman who lives in your neighborhood.
2. Try to avoid making it with a girl in the office. The office grapevine could reach all the way to your wife's ears.
3. Confine your extracurricular love-making to weekdays. Nothing will make your wife more suspicious than two or three "emergency weekend business trips."
4. Double-check for such telltale signs as lipstick on your collar and underclothing or a woman's hair on your jacket. Women—wives especially—are born detectives and they'll notice even the slightest details that could give you away.
5. When you leave for the evening, never tell your wife you're going to a place where she could check up on you. For example, don't tell her that you're going to a friend's house. One phone call by your wife and it's all over.
6. Never take your date to a restaurant or bar that your friends and neighbors frequent.
7. Never tell your paramour that you plan to divorce your wife and marry her. She could "help" things along a little by seeing to it that your wife happens to find out about your affair.

8. If you're paying rent or buying clothes and presents for your illicit partner in pleasure, pay cash. Those signed checks and credit card slips could be very incriminating.

9. Never bring your girl friend home when your wife is away. Neighbors have a way of looking out of windows.

If you are planning on having an affair there is one thing that you should remember. Your wife has the same sexual right as you do. The old double standard is rapidly being trampled by the new attitude of sexual freedom for both sexes. It's not uncommon for a wife to learn that her husband is being unfaithful and not to say anything about it. Instead she finds herself a boy friend. But this really shouldn't bother you. If you're a truly erotic husband, she'll have her fling and come back.

CHAPTER EIGHTEEN

Where and How to Meet Women

WE MEN are very lucky because we happen to be in relatively short supply. Women outnumber us by about 3 percent and that means while every guy can have a girl, not every girl can have a man. And simple economics tells us that when demand (there's always a demand for eligible men) exceeds supply, the supplier can hold out for the best deal. All this is a roundabout way of saying that there's no need for a halfway decent guy to be desperate for a woman and lunge at the first chick who happens to come down the pike. Most men, and *especially* erotic men, can afford to bide their time and wait for women who come closest to their ideals. There's a big selection of women and if a guy is patient he can find just what he wants. Remember, on the whole chicks need you more than you need them.

Although there are more women than men, I've heard many guys complain that they don't know where to go to find decent chicks. The severity of this problem depends on where you happen to be.

For an extreme example, when I was in basic training it got so bad that I started picturing my sergeant in long hair and a mini-skirt. But on the other hand, if you live in a city, a large town or within commuting distance of any population center, there's bound to be more than enough women for any guy. A bit later on I'm going to mention some of my favorite hunting grounds, but first I'd like to talk about where *not* to go to meet girls.

On the very top of my list of places to avoid when searching out the fair sex is a computer dating service, and I say this out of experience. A few years ago a buddy of mine showed up at the office one morning with a couple of application forms for a computer dating service. As a joke, he suggested that we fill them out and send them to the service along with the ten dollar fee. For our ten bucks we were guaranteed three telephone numbers of women who were electronically matched to the information we had indicated on the application. My friend got his reply first and called the girl who was number one on the list. When he spoke to her over the phone she sounded nice, but when he saw her in person she turned out to be a horror. Now I know it's not right to judge people by their appearances, but even being nice has its limits. This chick was easily fifty pounds overweight, kind of sloppy in her appearance and an incessant giggler. Being a gentleman, my friend suppressed his first impulse to turn tail and run and decided to take her to a movie. That way he didn't have to look at her.

Needless to say, he never took her out again nor did he bother calling the other two names on the list.

It wasn't long after his experience that I received my list of three names. The first girl I called quizzed me for about an hour about my job, my looks, my education and just about every other fact of my life. I felt as though I was going through a CIA security check rather than arranging a date. I hung up the phone without asking her out. The second girl I called was pleasant sounding on the phone and, surprisingly, relatively good looking in person. However, she turned out to be the most frigid female I'd ever met. A limp handshake, a peck on the cheek and an "I've had a wonderful evening" was all I got when I took her home. She was not for yours truly. I tore up the list with the remaining names. So much for my experience with computer dating.

Singles' weekends aren't much better. I had the misfortune to go on a three-day skiing trip with a group of the most lifeless men and women I've ever had the misfortune to meet. The group was divided into two types: the men whose wallets were loaded with condoms and whose minds were filled with thoughts of getting laid, and the women whose suitcases were probably packed with wedding gowns and whose eyes were alert for prospective marriage partners. The trip ended without one guy—myself included—getting laid and without one girl finding "Mr. Wonderful." On the second day of the trip I got to wishing I'd break a leg on the slopes so that the ambulance would take me to some place a little cheerier than the ski lodge . . . like a hospital for instance.

Third on my list of ways not to meet women is accepting blind dates from well-meaning relatives or your mother's friends. Now I'm not knocking blind dates in general. If a friend of yours, whose judgment and taste you can trust, offers you a blind date you'd probably do well to accept it. But if some old aunt says "I've got a girl for you," tell her that your reserve unit was just called up and you're leaving for Greenland tomorrow.

And my last suggestion for places to avoid when looking for swinging chicks is church dances, socials and picnics. If your mind is set on finding a girl who can appreciate an erotic man, you'd better do your looking is less wholesome places. Church-type chicks usually don't swing the way you do.

Now that we've covered the places not to look, let's talk about places where the pickings are apt to be a lot better. The first approach to successful woman-hunting is the shotgun approach. That is, covering all the places that hip girls are known to frequent.

Singles bars are good places to start. Since it has become respectable for women to allow themselves to be "picked up" in bars, you'll probably find a lot of girls who are out for the same kind of good time that you are. Of course, these singles spots will have their fair share of prudes in sexpot's clothing and pseudo-swingers who'll turn you on with subtle hints about their sex lives and then turn you off with "What kind of girl do you think I am?" when you've got them alone. But you've got to be able to adjust your erotic radar to pick out the legitimate swingers from the phonies. And all that takes is a little practice on your part.

The shotgun approach has taken me to many other places. The best among them have been resort areas during the Christmas and Easter holidays, rock festivals, discotheques, cocktail parties, college dances and literally any other place where there was sure to be a large gathering of people. Remember when you use the shotgun approach, the more girls there are in any one place the greater is your probability of finding one you'll like and who will like you.

Now some advice for men with more specific tastes in women, men who know almost exactly what they want. This is the specific approach, and works like this. If you have special interests and you want to find a companion who shares those interests, simply go to the places where such women are likely to be. For example, I'm a nut for modern art and I've found that on Sundays the Guggenheim Museum and the Museum of Modern Art, both in New York City, not only have interesting *objets d'art* hanging on the walls but they also have some walking around. And the beauty of it is that starting a conversation with a girl in an art museum is one of the easiest things to do. Simply pass a comment on the painting and in no time you're talking about lots of other things, like where to go for dinner. If art doesn't happen to be your thing, maybe politics or social issues are. The logical thing to do then is to go to a rally, a protest or a mass march. I'm not really into politics myself, but during the few occasions when I did protest something or rally in favor of a particular political issue I almost always managed to leave the demonstration with someone. By the same token if your bag is music, concerts have their female devotees. Or if you're the outdoor type, try a skating rink or ski lodge. I think you've got the idea. Go where your favorite kind of action is and you're sure to find a girl there who'll share it with you.

One final note on where to meet girls. When you get wherever your search takes you, don't stand around and "survey the field" before you make your move. There are a lot of guys who also have their eyes out for a good thing and you'd better act first if you don't want the leftovers. Here are some suggestions that I've found useful at parties, dances, or singles spots:

1. Stand as close to the door as possible so that you can have the first look at who's coming in.

2. As soon as you spot a girl you think might be worth your while, scoot over to the bar—which will probably be the first place she'll go—offer her a drink and start a conversation.

3. If she doesn't go to the bar or refreshment table, wait a minute or two for her to start talking to someone and then immediately move into the con-

versation. But don't wait too long to do this because she might just become too interested in what the other guy is saying.

This brings us to the next problem: "How do you approach a girl?" For me this was always more difficult than finding them. Practically all my adult life I've been surrounded by women, but I never used to know how to strike up a conversation with a woman without being clumsy. I guess I was just shy. But I learned that I wasn't the only man with this problem and I figured that if other men could overcome their shyness, so could I.

The way I did it was to rehearse a few opening lines. Not whole speeches, but just a few words to break the ice and get me going. Interestingly enough, the openers that have been most successful for me are the simple and direct ones like, "Hi, do you mind if I join you?" or "Would you like to dance?" Depending on the situations in which you meet women, other successful ice breakers are:

At political rallies—"I'm really surprised that all these people turned out. I didn't think it had aroused so much interest."

At a party given by a friend—"You must be a new addition to the old gang. I don't think I've ever met you here before."

At a large party where no one knows anyone—"Hi. You seem to be as lost as I am."

The trick is to be direct and avoid the cliches like, "Haven't I met you somewhere before?" Such worn-out lines are sure to earn you a cold shoulder. Another thing to avoid are the lines that obviously sound like cheap come-ons. "Where have you been all my life?" is one, and "I was about to leave, but since you've walked in I think I'm going to stay" is another. Chicks today are sophisticated and they appreciate straightforward honesty rather than gratuitous compliments.

After you've fired your opening shot, don't ruin your efforts with dull and uninspired follow-up conversation like playing "Who Do You Know?" or commenting about the weather. Talk about things you suspect will interest the both of you. Politics, music, fashions, women's lib, anything that lights a spark of interest in her eyes. I've found that astrology is of great interest to many chicks. Asking about a girl's birth sign and then commenting about the characteristics of Virgos, Taureans or whatever sign she was born under provides a lively few minutes of good small talk. Of course, you should mention your sign and talk about that.

So far you've done most of the talking, and that can be dangerous. Part of your approach to women must take into consideration the fact that they've got something to say. So don't monopolize the conversation. Provide them with enough openings so they'll feel at ease talking with you. Chances are that many girls you'll meet are as shy as you are and by allowing them to express themselves freely, they'll gradually overcome their shyness and you'll both get to know each other much better.

Once you've gotten to know a chick you may find that you don't go for her and that you'd rather spend your time looking for someone more to your liking. The trick now is to gradually ease yourself away from her. At large parties, music festivals or crowded parties, this is easy. Just excuse yourself and get lost in the crowd. In a few minutes she'll get the idea that you're not coming back and feel free to start talking to another guy. But in closer quarters like small gatherings, slipping away is not quite so easy. One way to free yourself without being discourteous is to call over a friend, introduce the girl to him and then clam up while they talk. After a few minutes you can walk away and no one will miss you. Another way is to say, "We've been ignoring the other guests," and direct your private conversation to the other people at the party. Once she's involved with them, you can try another opening line with another girl.

The opportunities and places for meeting chicks are only as limited as your ability to find them. Women are no longer cloistered in the home under the protective eyes of their parents; they're at parties, bars, hotels, resorts, museums, concerts and even right there in your office. In fact, almost any place you look you're bound to see lots of eligible females. And there is no insurmountable barrier between you and them. They want to meet you, they want to know you better and many of them want to make love to you if you'll just give them the opportunity. I don't care if you've flopped miserably before when it came to meeting women, you're an erotic man now and there's no reason in the world why, with just a little effort, you can't have the pick of the crop.

CHAPTER NINETEEN

Female Fantasies

EVERY ONE of us leads a double sex life, one real and one imagined. More often than not the fantasy sex life is much more exciting and fulfilling than the one we actually experience. The thousands of books about romance, the current vogue of "anything goes" films and controversial nudity on the stage all represent the attempts of authors and producers to cash in on our erotic dreams by making them come alive, at least for a moment, on the screen, the stage and in print. I'm convinced that almost every red-blooded young man or young woman wishes at one time or another that they could trade places, even for a day, with the romantic and sexually desirable heroes and heroines we read about or watch in the theater. In the past this wish would probably have been dismissed as a pipe dream, but today the sexual revolution has removed many of the old sexual taboos and placed sexual fantasies well within the reach of most people.

Although men tend to have a greater number of

sexual fantasies than women, women do nonetheless have their romantic and erotic dreams. And being an erotic man means being the answer to a woman's dream. If you could look into a chick's head and find out what she secretly desires the most from love-making and if you were able to satisfy these desires, you could go a long way toward improving both your girl's sex life as well as your own. Well, my friend, you can do exactly that, and I'm going to tell you how. I've done a little psychological detective work and asked chicks about their sexual fantasies. The result of my sleuthing was a very interesting and highly useful list of erotic games that women like to play.

THE SEX GODDESS FANTASY

Every woman with even the slightest bit of sensuality in her veins has, at one time or another thought of herself as a seductive and irresistible sex goddess with men literally fighting each other just to be with her. You can help this fantasy by suggesting in small ways that you are aware of your girl's qualities as a sexually sensational woman. Buy her sexy black underwear, revealing see-through nightgowns and lacy negligees. She'll appreciate these gifts as acknowledgments of her desirability, and when she wears them she'll be more sexy *and* she'll also feel the desire to live up to her image as a sex goddess.

Part of this fantasy is what I call the "stripper wish." That is, I've found that many, many women think of a strip teaser as a symbol of female seductiveness. And though chicks are hesitant to admit it, they'd probably like to do a sexy bump and grind while slowly peeling off their clothing as the men in the audience perspire and gape longingly at her. On several occasions I've been with girls who did reveal this hidden desire by turning up the stereo and going into a stripper routine that made Gypsy Rose Lee look like she was doing a tap dance at an elementary school assembly program. These chicks were the exception. But you can bring out the exhibitionist in your girl by dropping several hints. For example, buy her a copy of *How to Strip for Your Husband,* a paperback that offers a cram course in "taking it all off." Another way is buy her stripper clothes—a G-string and pasties— as a gag. You both may laugh at first, but don't be too surprised if she just decides to put them to use.

THE RAPE FANTASY

Sigmund Freud identified masochism as the female mode of sexual enjoyment and sadism as the male vehicle of erotic expression. In our culture women have things done to them sexually, while men are the doers. With this in mind, it's not strange that women often dream or fantasize situations in which they are being forced to make love against their wills, or in other words, being raped. This doesn't mean that I'm telling you to go out and rape a strange woman in order to prove you're an erotic man. That could get you into a bit of trouble. What I am saying is that sometimes when your girl says, "I'm not in the mood tonight," she's really saying, "Make me make love to you." Let me tell you a little story in this regard. Just recently I was seeing a girl whose sexual moods changed from hour to hour. At one moment there was nothing she wanted more than to climb into the sack, and then a moment later she was as cold as a snow-woman. I don't have to tell you how annoying this can be. So one time I just ignored her protests and went ahead and pulled her to the bed, took off her clothes and made love to her. It didn't take more than five minutes for her to warm up and respond to me. Later she told me that there was something exciting about what I did. She said, and I quote, "It was al-most like being raped."

THE BONDAGE FANTASY

Directly related to the Rape Fantasy is the Bondage Fantasy, the secret wish that certain women have to be tied to a bed or chair while men take liberties with them. This again represents the passive and masochis-tic nature of female sexuality. Although bondage is considered a perversion, it does have an increasing number of devotees, especially among certain way-out people who see nothing wrong with exotic sexual ex-perimentation. I myself wouldn't recommend that you suggest bondage to your girl—if she's not hip to this form of love-making she's liable to think you've gone bananas. But if a girl suggests it, I see no reason why you shouldn't let her have her desire. I've done it a few times and it's really quite interesting.

THE BABY DOLL FANTASY

Even in this modern day and age of women's libera-tion, many chicks still like to be pampered and made to feel ultra-feminine. They dream of men who shower them with silly gifts, treat them like fragile porcelain dolls and cater to their whims. I myself don't recom-mend this as a steady diet; it does become a drag after awhile and it also tends to make chicks too de-pendent on you. But once in awhile you'd be surprised at how much a girl will appreciate being treated this way. It helps her feel more like a woman and it makes you feel more like a man. And that is very important now that we are moving toward unisexualism, seeing the tendency of males and females to dress, look, think and act alike. A slight detour into the past helps to re-establish the best aspects of the traditional male-female relationship.

These are the fantasies that the women I spoke to revealed to me, and I suspect that they are shared by many women. However, your girl may have her own thing that she dreams about and wishes for and if you're clever enough to get her to tell you about it, you'll be in a better position to make her sexual dreams a reality. By the way, it wouldn't be a bad idea at all for you to confide your secret fantasies to her. Then she'll know what to do to make your fantasies more than a pipe dream.

CHAPTER TWENTY

Love and the Erotic Man

THROUGHOUT THIS book I've referred to intercourse as "making love" or as "love-making." Well, those are not really accurate terms to describe the physical union of a man and a woman. Making love, in the truest sense, is a lot more than merely getting laid. Both you and I know that a guy can make it with a chick, enjoy the action and even come back for a repeat performance without having any deep feelings that even remotely approach love for his bed partner. I'm not a romantic idealist who says that intercourse can't be enjoyable or satisfying unless there is an interchange of emotion between man and woman, because it can. Sex without love is far from impossible. However, I will say this—and I don't think anyone will dispute me—love can and does make sex a more complete experience, involving not only your genitals, but your emotions, mind and spirit as well.

Since I've become aware of my ability to please women and make them respond to me sexually, I've had many more erotic relationships with women than

I can accurately remember. Sometimes they were one-night stands, other times they were brief but red-hot affairs, and still on other occasions I stayed around a bit longer than I had planned because I discovered that a certain woman was more than a good partner; that she was exciting as a person, that she and I had ideas in common, and that I felt something for her that went beyond physical attraction. I guess you can say that once in awhile I did indeed fall in love. I don't consider myself the marrying type, at least not yet. There are too many things I want to do and see before I settle down. But that doesn't mean that I expect to spend all of my life jumping from one chick's bedroom to another. And it also doesn't mean that I'm incapable of falling in love with one woman for a little while or perhaps for longer than a little while if I find one woman so extraordinary that I'd be a fool to give her up. What I'm getting at is this: just as an erotic man must know how to make love, he must also know how to recognize love and to return it. Being unable to share a genuine love relationship with a woman makes a guy *unerotic,* he becomes nothing more than a stud; a body and mind ruled by an erection.

There's no doubt about it, the meaning of "love" is difficult, if not impossible for people to agree upon. And there are probably as many good definitions of love as there are people who attempt to define it. But if you've liked what I've said so far about improving the physical quality of your relationships with women, perhaps you'll also like what I've got to say about improving the psychological and spiritual quality of your relationships with the fair sex. In other words, you may like my feelings about love.

Love can be selfish or altruistic; wise or blind; or love can be a bartered agreement. When it comes to picking the type of love you want, you pay your money and take your choice. My choice is a love relationship that is altruistic and wise.

Sharing an altruistic love with a chick means that you and she merge almost as one person. Her problems become yours and yours, hers. You find yourself doing things for her because you want to do them and not because you expect anything in return. And you don't keep a tally sheet as to who does more for whom. Altruistic love means you take what she has to give, and you give her all you can and neither of you asks for more. When you make love to each other, the experience involves a total giving, and her sexual pleasure becomes an important part of your erotic enjoyment. But even with all the mutual feelings and oneness that you share, altruistic love doesn't stifle your individual personalities. There is a respect for the differences in temperament and these differences draw you closer together.

Loving wisely, as I see it, means that love *doesn't* dominate your every thought. Schoolboys and Victorian poets talk about a love so overwhelming that they become incapable of thinking about anything else except the person they love. But this is more infatuation than love. Loving wisely also means that you are aware of the faults in your girl's character—

no one is perfect. And it also means that you're aware of the problems that exist in all relationships between men and women. This awareness keeps you from pretending that everything is wonderful all the time, thereby saving you disillusionment and disappointment when certain problems cannot be ignored. A wise love also involves a realistic expectation of what love can and cannot do. If you think that merely being in love will make an ugly world go away, it won't. If you believe that love is unalterable and that it will always be as romantic as it was when you first met your girl, you're in for a disappointment. A wise lover knows that love is dynamic because it changes as two people mature together. Loving wisely means accepting rather than fighting these changes.

That's what I expect of love, but other people expect different things. Let's take a look at some other kinds of love and some feelings that some people confuse with love.

Selfish love is more or less the opposite of altruistic love. A man who loves selfishly wants his chick to do almost everything for him while he gives her little in return. He wants her to be ready to go places when he's ready, but sees nothing wrong in disappointing her. He demands faithfulness from his woman while he has a good time being a sexual butterfly. And in bed he makes great sexual demands on his chick so that his physical satisfaction is guaranteed and only reluctantly does a few things that she likes. Being a selfish lover is, in my book, the same thing as being a lousy lover. After awhile, a one-sided erotic affair gets rather dull and unexciting for a woman, and chances are that she'll wise up and look for a man who believes that sex involves a little more give-and-take.

Finally, being a selfish lover means using a woman to compensate for inadequacies real or imagined, that a man may have. Some guys dominate and abuse their women because they themselves are dominated and abused in the outside world. Still other guys need women who will reaffirm their faltering masculine image. By using a woman sexually, by having a chick act virtually as their slave, these guys selfishly exploit the love a woman may feel for them and turn it into the ego trip they need to feel more like men. But I've found that men who are selfish in this way are really not men at all. They're playing a part and doing a very bad job of it.

Bartered love is something like selfish love except that it involves a bit more give-and-take. A bartered relationship usually means a conditional type of love in which a man and woman agree to give each other what they want. For example, certain guys do not want to give up their exciting sex lives by settling down with one woman. But, on the other hand, they do want children, a home and a woman who can be a charming hostess for their business clients. And there are some women who want the financial security of marriage, the emotional security of children and the social security of at least a part-time husband to take them out once in awhile. Such men and women are meant for each other, and they enter a marriage of convenience. He agrees to give his wife the security and prestige she seeks, and she agrees to give him the home and children he wants—just as long as he is discreet about his extramarital affairs and avoids creating a scandal. Of course, there are many other types of bartered relationships, but this example should suffice to get the message across. The problem with bartered love is that frequently one or the other partner doesn't live up to the agreement and then things begin to fall apart. The sad fact is that conditional love doesn't come with an unconditional guarantee.

Blind love is the worst kind of love. To my way of thinking, love should be as realistic as people's emotions allow. But blind love doesn't permit reality to influence a man's feelings about a particular woman. Blind love glosses over obvious problems in a man-woman relationship and pretends they don't exist. Severe faults in a woman's character or personality are disregarded or treated as things that will disappear in time. But problems in the relationship and faults of character don't vanish by wishing them away, they endure and then suddenly appear so strongly and obviously that they can't be ignored any longer. At this point disillusionment sets in and eats away at whatever foundation the love relationship had. This myopic approach to love generally ends with a guy hating himself for having allowed himself to make such a foolish choice and he also often hates his former lover because he feels that she deceived him by letting him down. But this is self-deception and a man who falls in love blindly has no one but himself to blame for the inevitable unfortunate consequences. His only hope is that whatever heartaches his foolish love caused him will make him a little bit more aware and clearsighted the next time he decides to fall in love.

Blind love can, and generally does, arise from three seemingly harmless situations: infatuation, impulse and desire. I'm sure you remember when, sometime in early adolescence, you suddenly realized that girls were good for something other than taunting or throwing rocks at. That was the time of your first infatuation. The object of your affections was probably a girl who sat next to you in school and whom you passed notes to. She may have had braces on her teeth and freckles all over her face, but that didn't matter. You were in love for the first time and you were blind to her faults. Then, as your taste in women became somewhat more sophisticated, you probably found what you thought was the "ideal chick" and again infatuation hit you like a lead weight. That was okay then, and it was good experience. A carefree and exciting process was going on. You were maturing sexually and so was she. I remember several girls I was infatuated with when I was in high school and college. However, I didn't let these infatuations go on for too long before asking myself, "Is this really the girl I want?" and "Am I ready to be serious?" The answer to both these questions was always no, and these affairs came to an end. I was lucky. I know many guys who blindly followed their infatuations down the aisle and then realized that they had made a terrible mistake. They really didn't know the chicks they had married. And they hadn't realized exactly what marriage meant. It's serious business, too serious to enter with your eyes closed. Of course, infatuation can turn to love, but that happens when reality enters a relationship and undue romanticism leaves.

Impulse and desire have their place in the sex life of an erotic man. There are times when a certain girl suddenly appears and acts as a catalyst for your sexual chemistry. There's something about her; the way she looks, the clothes she wears or a teasing quality in her personality that makes you want to make love to her. At that moment you see her not as a person but as a sex object. Your desire runs high and you both find that you share an impulse to make passionate love. Well, that's cool. There's absolutely nothing wrong with giving your impulses a free run, just so long as you know when to pull in the reins. Sex may be enough to start a relationship, but it sure as hell isn't enough to sustain it. If you've got nothing in common with a girl except a mutual desire for some heavy balling, then enjoy it while it lasts and say good-bye before you become too involved.

Love, real love that is, makes certain requirements of you, and the two most important are that you respect yourself and the woman you think you've fallen for. It's not a very profound thing to say, but it is nonetheless true that you really can't love someone unless you first love yourself. By loving yourself, I definitely don't mean being an egomaniac whose every waking moment is devoted to self-adoration. Guys like that really turn chicks off. They're so involved with themselves that they are apt to be thoughtless, selfish and often unable to feel love for anyone but themselves. What self-love does mean is that you are aware of who you are and what you are and that you're capable of accepting yourself for both your good points and your bad ones as well. Pretending to be something you're not or deluding yourself into believing that you're as near perfect as any one human can be is the first step to creating emotional hang-ups —hang-ups that act as barriers to erotic gratification, because your preoccupation with fooling yourself and your chick doesn't allow you to relax enough to enjoy sex.

Self-love and self-respect also mean that you won't allow yourself to become a doormat for women, and that you don't become a tool that a girl can use in any way she pleases. Too many guys think they are showing love by doing whatever their girls want them to do, by giving in to their every whim and by abandoning their personal preferences and adopting a life style set for them by their women. This is a very foolish thing to do. Girls are human beings and human beings just naturally take advantage of people who are too nice. Any guy who doesn't display a reasonable amount of self-assertion is not going to win respect from his woman. Eventually he will lose her love. To be an erotic man you must strike a balance between being an overly dominating guy who thinks that even the slightest concession to a woman is a form of castration and being a Johnny-on-the-spot whenever she snaps her fingers. Self-love allows you to be an erotic man because it gives you enough pride to maintain your masculine image to yourself and your woman and at the same time it helps to learn how to yield to a woman without feeling that your maleness is in jeopardy.

I've mentioned above that love requires you to have a respect for the woman you feel strongly about, and this is essential. If you are using a chick for what you can get in the way of sex, if you think of her as a nice convenience to have around, and if you see her as being interchangeable with other girls you know, then you don't respect her feelings, her individuality, and you definitely don't love her. But if you are aware of her feelings and emotions and guard against hurting them, if you consider her likes and dislikes as being as valid as your own, and if you see in her what you've never seen in another female, then you respect her as a human being. And from that respect love can grow.

There is one thing I would like to clear up in regard to this idea of respecting women. I've heard a lot of guys say, "I'd like to go to bed with my girl, but I respect her too much to really try anything." Men who say this are victims of the moribund idea of chivalry. They believe that by not going to bed with a woman they love they are indicating respect. Hogwash! If you love and respect a woman, you want to share all kinds of beautiful things with her. And what's more beautiful than making love? What these knights in outdated armor are really saying is that they think sex is dirty and they don't want to risk deflowering their virginal princesses. I really don't think these men are showing respect as much as they are showing their own pruduish attitudes about sex. *Prudes cannot be erotic men!*

Well, there you have it. That's my personal philosophy on love. Take it for what it's worth to you. If I've answered some question you may have had about sex and love, good. If I've made you think about the emotional relationship you now have with a woman, that's even better. And if I've left you totally unimpressed with my views on love, I won't take it as a personal insult. You've got your thing and I've got mine. But there is one thing we can all agree upon, and that is something I said earlier: Without love, sex is an exercise that can be physically enjoyable. But with love, even if it's only a momentary exchange of emotions and understanding, sex can be a totally fulfilling experience. And one of the secrets of being an erotic man is to try to choose a girl whom you can feel love for—even if it's just a slight amount of love. If you do, you will be a much better lover. That much I can personally guarantee.

CHAPTER TWENTY-ONE

The Rest Is Up to You

WELL, BUDDY, now you know everything that I know about being an erotic man, the rest is up to you. I can only tell you what's worked for me. Now you have to make it work for yourself. It only takes a little self-confidence, imagination and practice.

Oh, sure, you're bound to come across some chicks who won't dig you; you'll find yourself in bed with a semi-prude who turns up her nose at oral sex; and you'll frustrate yourself trying to elicit an orgasm from some frigid female. But that's the breaks of the game. Being an erotic man doesn't mean you'll have a 100 percent fantastic sex life. No one except a liar would ever say that he's made it with every chick he took out or experienced an orgasm every time he made love. However, being an erotic man *does* mean that you'll do a lot better with chicks than you used to.

At the risk of sounding like a coach for the Sexual Olympics, let me offer you this little pep talk. If a chick rejects you, don't get bitter and curl up inside your shell. Pick up your marbles and play somewhere else. If you can't seem to get a particular woman excited, just think to yourself that it could be her and not you who's sexually deficient. And if a chick puts you down for not being sensational in bed, don't give up. Ask her out again, and this time pull out all the stops and let her have it with everything you know. You're bound to come up with the thing that turns her on.

That's about all for now. I've got to turn off my electric typewriter and get ready for my date tonight. Her name is Cheryl and she's a great-looking photographer's model. She goes wild for "French-style" lovemaking, she gives incredible massages, and once in awhile she teaches *me* a new thing or two. Cheryl invited me over to her house for dinner tonight, and guess what I'm having for dessert.

OTHER AWARD BOOKS
YOU'LL BE SURE TO ENJOY

OTHER AWARD BOOKS
YOU'LL BE SURE TO ENJOY

OTHER AWARD BOOKS
YOU'LL BE SURE TO ENJOY

SOUL SISTERS   Joan Blair
Swinging from chic East Side bars to Harlem, three young and
beautiful black girls go for a piece of the action in the white
world of money and success.   A666—75¢

THE BUYERS   Jack Martin Oppenheim
The big new novel about Seventh Avenue's sex-and-fashion
jungle—where decisions made at the top are often determined
by what goes on behind the racks.   A683—95¢

THE RUNNING MAN   W.A. Harbinson
He lived off the human flotsam of the white world—drifters,
prostitutes, and failures—and he made Whitey pay . . . but one
day he went too far . . . much too far . .   A603—60¢

THE DOOMSDAY COMMITTEE   Richard Gallagher
A novel of gripping terror and suspense that explores what
happens when an army of seething militants captures an Ameri-
can city—black-power style!   A670—75¢

THE FARM   Clarence L. Cooper, Jr.
"*The Farm* portrays a brutal and ugly world, but it conveys
vividly the sex-obsessed and angry mind of an alienated junkie."
—*Springfield Sun*   A659—75¢

OTHER AWARD BOOKS
YOU'LL BE SURE TO ENJOY

OTHER AWARD BOOKS
YOU'LL BE SURE TO ENJOY

OTHER AWARD BOOKS
YOU'LL BE SURE TO ENJOY

OTHER AWARD BOOKS
YOU'LL BE SURE TO ENJOY

ESP YOUR SIXTH SENSE   **Brad Steiger**
Do you have the power of Extra-Sensory Perception? You will be amazed at the answer in this up-to-the-minute probe of a subject as old as time itself!   A756—75¢

WISDOM OF THE ANCIENTS   **T. Lobsang Rampa**
For the first time, a spiritual leader explains, in simple language, the centuries-old Eastern truths which can lead to peace and contentment.   A768—75¢

SPIRITUAL HEALING   **John Pendragon & George Pasteur**
Here is the complete, totally amazing story of one of the world's great healers, George Pasteur—a man of miracles who has cured the "incurable."   A724—75¢

THE NATURE OF THE I CHING   **Charles Poncé**
Full instruction for the use of the fabled Oriental classic. An easy-to-follow guide to the most amazing method of foretelling the future known to man!   A547—75¢

COMPANIONS OF THE UNSEEN   **Paul Tabori**
The astounding stories of nine famous mediums, all subjects of scientific investigation, which will shock you as they shocked the experts!   A664—75¢

THE SKY PEOPLE   **Brinsley Le Poer Trench**
In this astounding but scholarly book you will find proof that visitors from other planets exist—and that they are among us now!   A706—75¢

HANDWRITING GUIDE TO LOVE & SEX   Dorothy Sara
Learn the simple art of handwriting analysis which can reveal
all the hidden personality traits of the man or woman in your life!
Fully illustrated   A722—95¢

THE BIG ANSWER BOOK ABOUT SEX   Dr. Paul J. Gillette
Here in *frank, explicit* language are all the sex questions you
ever had—answered! With a special introduction by Dr. Albert
Ellis.   A669—95¢

HORIZONTAL EXERCISES   Robert L. Rowan, M.D.
A physician's complete sexual-sensitivity program for men in
their middle and later years. Learn how to be sexually active all
your life!   A718—95¢

**THE LAYMAN'S EXPLANATION OF HUMAN
SEXUAL INADEQUACY**   Edited by Dr. Paul J. Gillette
A close look at the *second* Masters-and-Johnson report. It offers
the key to eliminating sexual problems.   A690—95¢